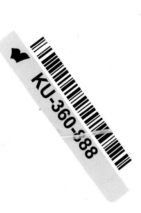

Radiographic Positioning

For Elsevier:

Commissioning Editor: Dinah Thom
Development Editor: Catherine Jackson
Project Manager: Christine Johnston
Designer: Erik Bigland
Illustrator: Cactus
Illustration Manager: Merlyn Harvey
Photographers/photo editors: Ruth Sutherland, Calum Thomson

POCKETBOOK OF

Radiographic Positioning

THIRD EDITION

Ruth Sutherland DCR(R)

Radiographer, NHS Grampian, Aberdeen, UK
Formerly Lecturer at Robert Gordon University, Aberdeen, UK

Calum Thomson DCR(R) BSc

Superintendent Radiographer Orthopaedics, Glasgow Royal Infirmary,
Glasgow, UK
Formerly Lecturer at Robert Gordon University, Aberdeen, UK

Foreword by
Donald Graham MEd TDCR
Formerly Director of the Department of Radiography,
School of Health Sciences, Robert Gordon University, Aberdeen, UK

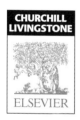

CHURCHILL
LIVINGSTONE

ELSEVIER

EDINBURGH LONDON NEW YORK OXFORD PHILADELPHIA ST LOUIS SYDNEY TORONTO 2007

CHURCHILL
LIVINGSTONE
ELSEVIER

© 1998, W.B. Saunders Company Ltd
© 2003, 2007, Elsevier Limited. All rights reserved.

First edition 1998
Second edition 2003
Third edition 2007
  Reprinted 2008, 2009

ISBN: 978 0 443 10330 8

British Library Cataloguing in Publication Data
A catalogue record for this book is available from the British Library.

Library of Congress Cataloging in Publication Data
A catalog record for this book is available from the Library of Congress.

Note

Knowledge and best practice in this field are constantly changing. As new research and experience broaden our knowledge, changes in practice, treatment and drug therapy may become necessary or appropriate. Readers are advised to check the most current information provided (i) on procedures featured or (ii) by the manufacturer of each product to be administered, to verify the recommended dose or formula, the method and duration of administration, and contraindications. It is the responsibility of the practitioner, relying on their own experience and knowledge of the patient, to make diagnoses, to determine dosages and the best treatment for each individual patient, and to take all appropriate safety precautions. To the fullest extent of the law, neither the Publisher nor the Authors assumes any liability for any injury and/or damage to persons or property arising out or related to any use of the material contained in this book.

The Publisher

CONTENTS

Chapter 1 – Upper Extremity

Chapter 2 – Shoulder Girdle

Chapter 3 – Thoracic Cage

Chapter 4 – Respiratory System

Chapter 5 – Abdominal Contents

Chapter 6 – Pelvis, Hip Joint and Upper Third of Femur

Chapter 7 – Lower Extremity

Chapter 8 – Vertebral Column

Chapter 9 – The Skull

Appendix

CD CONTENTS

The CD contains the positioning photographs and radiographs from the book, and allows them to be viewed in a larger, more realistic format.

In addition the CD contains:

'Assessing the image', which covers:

- a simplistic explanation of what makes up the various grey tones on the radiograph
- appearances of bone
- how a fracture can appear black or white
- bone development, radiographic appearances of child's hand and elbow
- ABCs – systematic approach to studying the radiograph/image
- Salter–Harris classification of epiphyseal fractures.

For each examination the CD includes:

- labelled radiographs
- alternative photographs/images to aid positioning
- extra information on technique
- information on assessment
- assessment/anatomy/centring tests.

The CD also includes a section on bare essentials of skull and facial bones trauma radiography (non-isocentric technique), and a number of examples of pathology for the student to study.

FOREWORD

A pocketbook has a number of advantages over a large textbook. These include the fact that: a pocketbook usually contains succinct information which is readily available to the reader; the material is logically laid out and the information is easy to find; and a pocketbook can be used by the student to find new information or by the professional as an *aide-mémoire*.

All of the above are true of the *Pocketbook of Radiographic Positioning*. It is written in a style which makes information gathering easy, and there is space within the text to allow the reader to customise the text for his or her individual use.

All textbooks to some extent are restricted when providing radiographs/photographs and as a consequence accurate interpretation is difficult. The authors have overcome this by an accompanying CD where the images can be seen in 'life-size' format as well as supplying a wealth of extra relevant material.

This CD is easy to negotiate and logical in its presentation. For each projection there is a detailed note of the technique with the opportunity to self-test to allow consolidation of essential information. There is also a self-test on the radiographic anatomy of the projection and sections dealing with pathology and medical terms and abbreviations. The CD allows for a larger format of image which is especially useful when demonstrating positioning of the structure and also in showing the radiographic appearances.

I feel that the combination of the pocketbook and the CD will prove popular with students, with radiographic assistants and with many radiographers as well. This enhances an already well-established learning facility, which will be well received by the profession.

Donald Graham

PREFACE

The *Pocketbook of Radiographic Positioning* and CD is intended primarily for the use of student radiographers, radiography assistant practitioners, newly qualified radiographers and clinical educators. Health professionals such as A and E nurses, extended scope practitioners and those involved in requesting X-ray examinations will also find the material of great use and interest.

The CD is new to this edition and contains material from the book and also other very useful information. One of the many purposes of the book and accompanying CD is to provide the information needed to help produce and maintain highly informed radiographers.

Radiographers are required to decipher and justify the request form, assess the patient, match the needs of the patient to the technique to be employed, reassure the patient, ensure that both IR(ME)R and ALARP regulations are adhered to, and finally assess the resultant 'diagnostic' image. All this has to be done in a few minutes in a quick, timely and professional manner. The resultant image can be measured, analysed and has to be of diagnostic quality; suboptimal images are rarely if ever acceptable. Radiographers' work is there for immediate scrutiny, sometimes by a multitude of onlookers – surgeons, nurses, doctors and radiologists. It must be at least 'adequate' and fit for purpose – they have one chance to get it right and cannot say come back in a week. However the radiograph, 'our work', can be reviewed many times for many years to come by everyone from patients to lawyers. So to all present and future multi-tasking radiographers well done and I hope the book and CD is a useful aid to your work 'under the microscope'.

The CD allows the images from the book, both photographs and radiographs, to be viewed in a much larger format. This format enables the images to be labelled, and in many cases extra positioning tips have been added.

In addition to the book contents there are:

- Extra photographs showing the positioning of the patient from a different aspect.
- Labelled radiographs with self-test function.
- General information on how to assess a radiograph.
- Radiographs with assessment lines and areas of interest highlighted.
- A section on A and E skull – non-isocentric technique.
- Examples of fractures and pathology for most sections.

The pathologies and fractures are included to allow the reader to assess the radiographic image and identify the 'abnormality'.

The **book** contains the basic skeletal and some soft tissue radiographic examinations. It is not intended to be a comprehensive textbook on radiographic positioning, more of an *aide-mémoire* in a pocket-sized form.

Included are the following:

- Patient position photographs – to support the text and to give greater emphasis to the patient's position.

- Appropriate radiographs to confirm that the required result of the examination has been achieved.

- Simple hints to aid positioning ✓.

- Some common errors to be avoided ✗.

- Indication of susceptible areas of trauma or pathology.

- Indication of some epiphysis calcification dates.

Excluded:

- Exposure factors. Specific exposure charts should be displayed in the appropriate imaging rooms. IR(ME)R (Ionising Radiation (Medical Exposure) Regulations) – *a small table has been included to record exposure factors/dose for each area.*

- Some skeletal examinations. Some examinations are now not recommended in consideration of the 'as low as reasonably practicable' (ALARP) principle.

- Specialised examinations such as computerised tomography (CT), magnetic resonance imaging (MRI), radionuclide imaging (RNI), ultrasound and fluoroscopy. This is due to the diversity of the protocols used. There are specific books written about these techniques that can be used for reference.

- Nomenclature, pads and sandbags. These may be absent from some of the photographs purely to aid visualisation of the image. The majority of patients do not need pads when imaged by a radiographer well practised in technique.

To conclude this preface it is important to mention that there are many ways to achieve the same result. Some radiographers prefer to move the patient, others to angle the tube. For a specific examination some departments will perhaps take three projections, others only two. Local protocols must be adhered to, and students and new members of staff should ensure that they become familiar with local techniques and protocols.

I would also like to pass on a comment from my tutor (Ted Foster) of many years ago who sadly is no longer with us:

'The patient is always central and should be treated with respect whatever the injury. We perhaps do not know all the detail: a badly injured leg from an RTA might appear very dramatic whilst the next patient with a crushed finger distal phalanx in comparison appears very slight. However, take the scenario nine months down the line: the leg is fully healed and the patient returned to his office work with no apparent disability, while the distal phalanx fracture has healed but the professional concert pianist is unable to work!'

Aberdeen and	Ruth Sutherland
Glasgow 2007	Calum Thomson

ACKNOWLEDGEMENTS

We would like to thank the Medical Director for NHS Grampian for granting permission to use anonymised digital images from the Trust and to thank Mark for supplying them. We would also like to thank Ann Helen (Bergen, Norway) for providing some of the digital images.

IMPORTANT CONSIDERATIONS

Purpose

This book is intended to be a quick reference guide and is essentially for use in the clinical environment.

Standard factors to be considered throughout

- Source to image distance (SID) will be 100 cm unless stated.
- Patient care must be maintained at all times.
- Radiation dose must be considered for all examinations in the form of accurate collimation, application of lead rubber aprons and shielding, good radiographic techniques and the choice of exposure factors to apply the ALARP principle.
- Nomenclature/immobilisation aids and use of split films should be made in accordance with National/Local protocols; the photographs in the book do not include these to allow better visualisation of the actual technique.
- Adherence to implementation of IR(ME)R 2000 Regulations.
- # – Fracture
- < – Less than
- > – Greater than.

RADIOGRAPHIC POSITIONING TERMINOLOGY

The anatomical position

- Subject facing forwards
- Body erect
- Arms and legs fully extended
- Palms of the hands are facing forwards and the feet are together

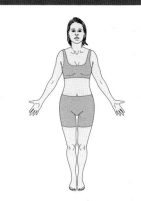

Median sagittal plane

- Passes vertically through the midline of the body dividing the body into a left and a right half in equal portions

Sagittal plane

- Any plane passing through the body parallel to the median sagittal plane

Coronal plane

- Passes vertically through the midline of the body dividing the body into an anterior and a posterior half in equal portions

Transverse plane

- Any plane passing through the body at right angles to the median sagittal plane dividing the body into a superior and inferior portion

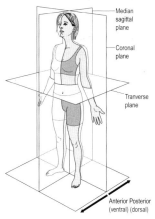

RADIOGRAPHIC PROJECTIONS

Anteroposterior (AP)

- Patient can be supine on the X-ray table or erect with back against the vertical stand. The central ray enters the front (anterior) and exits the back (posterior) surface of the body.

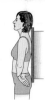

Posteroanterior (PA)

- Patient can be prone on the X-ray table or erect facing the vertical stand. The central ray enters the back (posterior) and exits the front (anterior) surface.

Lateral

- Patient can lie on either side on the X-ray table or erect with either side against the vertical stand. The projection is always named after the side of the body closest to the cassette.

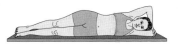

Left anterior oblique (LAO)

- Patient is erect or semi-prone. The *left* side of the body is closest to the cassette.

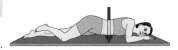

Right anterior oblique (RAO)

- Patient erect or semi-prone. The *right* side of the body is closest to the cassette.

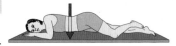

Left posterior oblique (LPO)

- Patient erect or semi-supine. The *left* side of the body is closest to the cassette.

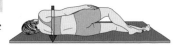

Right posterior oblique (RPO)

- Patient erect or semi-supine. The *right* side of the body is closest to the cassette.

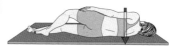

Dorsal decubitus

- Patient is supine on the X-ray table or trolley. The central ray enters from one side of the patient and exits from the opposite side.

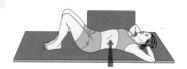

Ventral decubitus

- Patient is prone on the X-ray table or trolley. The central ray enters from one side of the patient and exits from the opposite side.

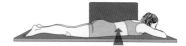

Lateral decubitus

- Patient lying on either side.

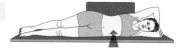

Left lateral decubitus

- Patient lying on the left side with the right side uppermost.

Right lateral decubitus

- Patient lying on their right side with the left side uppermost.

1 Upper Extremity

FINGERS

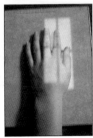 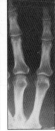

Projection: PA (DORSIPALMAR)
Centring Point: To the proximal interphalangeal joint

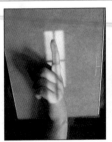 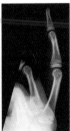 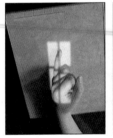 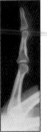

Second finger   **Fifth finger**

Projection: LATERAL
Centring Point: To the proximal interphalangeal joint

Points to consider

Technique

- ☑ Metacarpophalangeal joint *must* be included
- ☑ Always include another finger to aid identification
- ☑ AP – the fingers *must* be placed flat upon the cassette
- ☑ Lateral – non-opaque pad can be used to help extend the finger
- ☒ Lateral – trauma – try not to let the finger flex too much

kV	mAs	focus	film/screen	bucky	dose

Radiological assessment

☑ Avulsion #s are common – look for soft tissue swelling
☑ Mallet finger – direct blow plus avulsion of extensor tendon
☑ Dislocation – proximal interphalangeal joint – sporting injury
☑ Joint spaces should be uniform – approximately 1mm in width
☑ Transverse # – result of hyperextension of the finger

PA (dorsipalmar) – affected finger

- Patient seated, affected side towards the X-ray table
- Forearm placed on table
- Palmar aspect of fingers placed on the cassette
- Fingers extended and separated slightly

Collimation

To include: PROXIMALLY: Full length of metacarpal
               DISTALLY: Terminal phalanx
               LATERALLY: Soft tissue borders
   Include adjacent finger to aid identification

Lateral – index and middle fingers

- Hand rotated medially until the lateral aspect of the index finger is in contact with the cassette
- Index and middle fingers are extended and separated
- Remaining fingers are flexed
- Forearm may be raised on pads and supported – middle finger may be supported with a non-opaque pad

Lateral – little and ring fingers

- Hand rotated laterally so that the medial aspect of the little finger is in contact with the cassette
- Little and ring fingers are extended and separated
- Ring finger may be supported on a non-opaque pad and parallel to the cassette
- Remaining fingers are flexed

Collimation

To include: PROXIMALLY: Proximal phalanx
               DISTALLY: Terminal phalanx
               LATERALLY: Soft tissue borders

THUMB

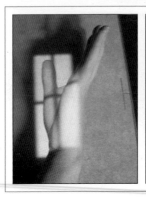 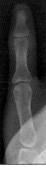

Projection: AP
Centring Point: To the metacarpophalangeal joint

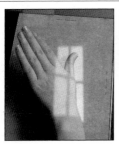 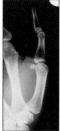

Projection: LATERAL
Centring Point: To the metacarpophalangeal joint

Points to consider

Technique

- ☑ AP – condyles must be equidistant from the cassette
- ☑ Lateral – condyles must be superimposed
- ☑ ?Trauma – consider alternative AP (trauma) projection
- ☒ Underpenetration of proximal thumb due to thenar pad

kV	mAs	focus	film/screen	bucky	dose

Radiological assessment

☑ Radiograph can appear normal – look for soft tissue swelling

☑ Avulsion #s may be present

☑ Bennett's # – # dislocation – result of forced abduction

☑ Skier's (gamekeeper's) thumb – acute sprain or rupture – ulnar collateral ligament

AP

- Patient seated, affected side towards the X-ray table
- Thumb, elbow and shoulder at the same height (desirable but not essential)
- The hand and forearm are extended
- Hand rotated medially so that the posterior aspect of the thumb is in contact with the cassette

Collimation

To include: PROXIMALLY: Carpometacarpal joint
DISTALLY: Terminal phalanx
LATERALLY: Soft tissue borders
MEDIALLY: Soft tissue borders

Lateral

- Patient seated
- Hand prone, the palm is then rotated medially and supported on a non-opaque pad until the thumb is lateral, fingers form fist to support position or use non-opaque pad where indicated
- Lateral aspect of the thumb is in contact with the cassette and is then slightly flexed

Collimation

To include: PROXIMALLY: Carpometacarpal joint
DISTALLY: Terminal phalanx
LATERALLY: Soft tissue borders
MEDIALLY: Soft tissue borders

THUMB

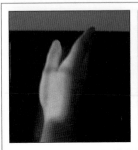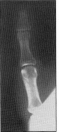

Projection: AP ALTERNATIVE POSITION (TRAUMA)
Centring Point: To the metacarpophalangeal joint

Points to consider

Technique

- ☑ Use if injury to base of first metacarpal is suspected
- ☑ Where indicated support the thumb on a non-opaque pad
- ☑ *Must* include the carpometacarpal joint
- ☑ Increase SID to reduce the magnification
- ☑ Thumb *must* be parallel to the cassette

Radiological assessment

- ☑ Check the first carpometacarpal joint is included
- ☒ A magnified image unless an increased SID is used
- ☒ Bennett's # – unlikely thumb will be parallel to the cassette

AP alternative position (trauma)

- Medial border of the hand, placed in contact with the cassette
- Palmar aspect 90°
- Thumb is extended and where indicated placed on a non-opaque pad

kV	mAs	focus	film/screen	bucky	dose

If the patient's thumb is in a cast, the patient standing often enables the thumb to be more easily placed parallel to the cassette.

Collimation

To include: PROXIMALLY: Carpometacarpal joint
               DISTALLY: Terminal phalanx
               LATERALLY: Soft tissue borders
               MEDIALLY: Soft tissue borders

HAND

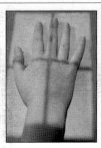 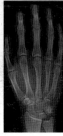

Projection: PA (DORSIPALMAR)

Centring Point: To the head of the third metacarpal

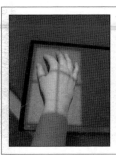 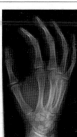

Projection: PA OBLIQUE

Centring Point: To the head of the third metacarpal

Points to consider

Technique

- ☑ Include the whole of the hand, including carpal bones and distal radius/ulna
- ☑ ?Injury confined to distal digit – limit image to that digit
- ☑ If you identify an injury – proceed to a lateral
- ☑ PA oblique – better general assessment if fingers parallel
- ☒ PA oblique – avoid over-rotation – obscure metacarpals

kV	mAs	focus	film/screen	bucky	dose

Radiological assessment

☑ #s metacarpal neck – usually the result of a direct blow

☑ Common site for #s – head of the fifth metacarpal – Boxer's #

☑ Look for vertical # through the base with dislocation of joint

☑ Secondary ossification centres appear at age 2–3 years

☒ PA poor at showing #s of the articular surface of the metacarpal heads

PA (dorsipalmar)

● Patient seated, affected side towards the X-ray table

● Palmar aspect placed on the cassette

● Fingers are extended and slightly separated

Collimation

To include: PROXIMALLY: Distal radius and ulna
DISTALLY: Terminal phalanx
LATERALLY: Soft tissue borders
MEDIALLY: Soft tissue borders

PA oblique

● From the PA position the hand is rotated onto the lateral side to form an angle of 45° and where indicated supported on a non-opaque pad

● Fingers slightly flexed and separated

● Fingertips in contact with the cassette

Collimation

To include: PROXIMALLY: Distal radius and ulna
DISTALLY: Terminal phalanx
LATERALLY: Soft tissue borders
MEDIALLY: Soft tissue borders

HAND

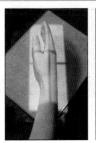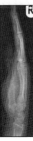

Projection: LATERAL

Centring Point: To the head of the second metacarpal

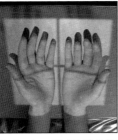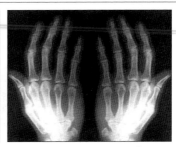

Projection: AP OBLIQUE (BALL CATCHER'S)

Centring Point: Midway between both hands at the level of the head of the fifth metacarpal

Points to consider

Technique

☑ Lateral – where indicated support the thumb on a non-opaque pad

☒ If not a true lateral – may result in missing a dislocation

☑ An increase in exposure of up to 5kV may be necessary

☑ Catcher's – obliquity – metacarpal heads *must* be free from superimposition

kV	mAs	focus	film/screen	bucky	dose

Radiological assessment

☑ Look for bone alignment – displacement and dislocation

☑ Look for # through the articular surface at the base of phalanx

☑ Check the base of the fourth and fifth metacarpals – dislocation is common

☑ Ball catcher's – look for early rheumatoid arthritis with loss of bony outline and associated demineralisation

Lateral

- From the oblique position the hand is rotated laterally so that the palmar aspect forms an angle of 90° to the cassette
- Fingers are extended and superimposed
- Thumb is extended away from the metacarpals and where indicated placed upon a non-opaque pad

Collimation

To include: PROXIMALLY: Distal radius and ulna
DISTALLY: Terminal phalanx
LATERALLY: Soft tissue borders

AP oblique (ball catcher's)

- Patient seated facing the X-ray table (use lead rubber gonad protection)
- Both forearms and hands are supinated
- Dorsa of both hands are in contact with the cassette and fifth metacarpals and phalanges are touching
- Hands are then internally rotated 45° as if to catch a ball
- Hands where indicated are supported in position with non-opaque pads

Collimation

To include both hands

WRIST

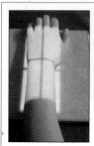 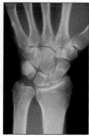

Projection: PA

Centring Point: Midway between the styloid processes

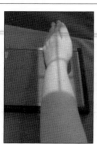 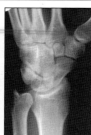

Projection: PA OBLIQUE

Centring Point: Midway between the styloid processes

Points to consider

Technique

☑ AP – elbow and wrist at the same level

☑ Is there ulnar deviation if a scaphoid # is suspected?

☑ Slightly curl fingers so that carpals are in contact with cassette

☑ Dry plaster of Paris cast increase 1 stud kV + 1 stud mAs

☑ Wet plaster of Paris cast increase 2 stud kV + 1 stud mAs

☑ Synthetic cast increase 1 stud mAs

☒ Be careful of abnormally thick plaster casts

kV	mAs	focus	film/screen	bucky	dose

Radiological assessment

✓ Colles' # – posterior displacement – most common in the elderly – displacement described as 'dinner fork' deformity

✓ Smith's # – anterior displacement – uncommon

✓ Epiphyses – radial appears in the second year and fuses in the 20th year – ulnar appears in the 8th year and fuses in the 20th year

PA

- Patient seated, affected side towards the X-ray table
- Elbow is flexed, wrist and forearm placed onto the cassette
- Fingers are slightly flexed to raise the hand and keep the wrist in contact with the cassette
- Styloid processes are equidistant from the cassette

PA oblique

- From the PA position the wrist is rotated laterally until the palmar aspect is approximately 45° to the cassette
- Where indicated a non-opaque pad is placed under the radial side of the wrist

Collimation

To include: PROXIMALLY: Lower third of radius and ulna
DISTALLY: Head of the metacarpals
LATERALLY: Soft tissue borders
MEDIALLY: Soft tissue borders

WRIST

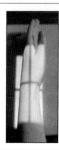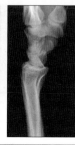

Projection: LATERAL

Centring Point: To the radial styloid process

Points to consider

Technique

- ☑ Styloid processes *must* be superimposed – rotate further 5°
- ☑ To achieve superimposition try extending the elbow
- ☑ Wrist and elbow should be at the same level
- ☑ Acute injury – horizontal beam will be necessary

Radiological assessment

- ☑ In children look for a slipped epiphysis
- ☑ Look for soft tissue swelling due to haemorrhage
- ☑ Commonest carpal dislocation – lunate dislocation due to forced dorsiflexion
- ☑ Triquetrum is the second commonest carpal bone to #
- ☑ In children – commonest # is the greenstick

Lateral

- Hand is rotated so that the palmar aspect is at 90° to the cassette
- Elbow is flexed
- Wrist may be rotated a further 5° posteriorly to superimpose the styloid processes
- Where indicated thumb is supported on a non-opaque pad

kV	mAs	focus	film/screen	bucky	dose

Collimation

To include: PROXIMALLY: Lower third of radius and ulna
DISTALLY: Head of the metacarpals
LATERALLY: Soft tissue borders
MEDIALLY: Soft tissue borders

SCAPHOID

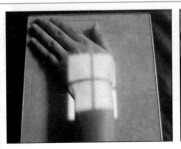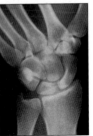

Projection: PA
Centring Point: Midway between the styloid processes

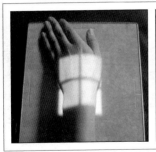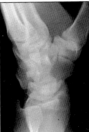

Projection: PA OBLIQUE
Centring Point: Midway between the styloid processes

Points to consider

Technique

☑ PA – ulnar deviation essential where injury will allow

☑ Fine focus is essential

☑ Long axis of the scaphoid should be parallel to the cassette

☑ Increase mAs slightly due to precise collimation

☒ *Do not* X-ray through plaster due to poor definition

kV	mAs	focus	film/screen	bucky	dose

Radiological assessment

☑ PA – the scaphoid and joint spaces should be demonstrated

☑ 80% of #s occur at the waist of the scaphoid and jeopardise blood supply to the proximal part

☑ Scaphoid # may not be evident for 5–10 days after injury – *must* have a follow-up examination

☑ # of the proximal pole of scaphoid – increased chance of avascular necrosis

☑ Look for reabsorption of bone on follow-up radiographs

PA

- Patient seated, affected side towards the X-ray table
- Elbow is flexed, wrist and forearm placed onto the cassette
- Fingers are slightly flexed to raise the hand and keep the wrist in contact with the cassette
- Styloid processes are equidistant from the cassette
- Ulnar deviation of the hand

PA oblique

- From the PA position the wrist is rotated laterally until the palmar aspect is approximately 30–45° to the cassette
- A non-opaque pad may assist with reducing motion but is not always necessary

Collimation

For maximum image resolution – collimate precisely to include the carpal bones

SCAPHOID

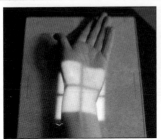 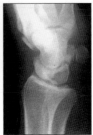

Projection: AP OBLIQUE

Centring Point: Midway between the styloid processes

Points to consider

Technique

☑ A slight over-rotation of the wrist will superimpose the styloid processes

☑ Minimise movement of the wrist as much as possible – move the wrist from the elbow and shoulder

☑ A kV increase will be required for the lateral projection

☑ Oblique – hand, where indicated support with non-opaque pads

Radiological assessment

☑ If intercarpal joints measure more than 2mm (adult) then suspect ligamentous injury

☑ 90% of carpal #s involve the scaphoid

☑ Lateral – most dislocations involve the lunate bone

☑ Oblique – pisiform and posterior triquetral should be visible

kV	mAs	focus	film/screen	bucky	dose

AP oblique

- From the lateral position the wrist is rotated a further 45° so that the palmar aspect of the hand is uppermost
- A non-opaque pad may be placed under the radial side of the wrist

Collimation

For maximum image resolution – collimate precisely to include the carpal bones
A coned down lateral wrist may be requested as part of a scaphoid series

SCAPHOID

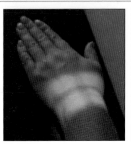 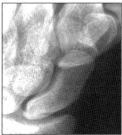

Projection: POSSIBLE SCAPHOID

Centring Point: To the scaphoid – just distal to the anatomical snuff box. Central ray 30° towards the elbow

Points to consider

Technique

- ☑ Ulnar deviation essential
- ☑ Slightly raised fingers are due to carpals in contact with cassette
- ☑ Angle the central ray 30° – check SID is still 100 cm
- ☒ Too much angle of central ray will distort the scaphoid
- ☒ Take care not to project the image off the cassette

Radiological assessment

- ☑ Separates the scaphoid from the carpal bones
- ☑ Exaggerates a # if present
- ☑ May require RNI if pain persists and X-rays show no abnormality
- ☒ Elongated projection – use as a supplementary projection only

Possible scaphoid fracture (alternative 'banana projection')

- Patient seated, affected side towards the table
- Elbow is flexed to 90°

kV	mAs	focus	film/screen	bucky	dose

- Ulnar deviation of the wrist
- Central ray 30° towards the elbow along the axis of the radius and ulna

Collimation

For maximum image resolution – collimate precisely to include the carpal bones

FOREARM

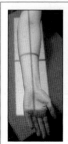 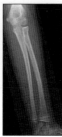

Projection: AP
Centring Point: To the middle of the forearm

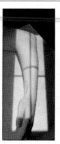 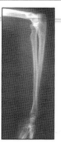 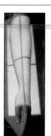 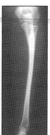

Projection: LATERAL 1   LATERAL 2
Centring Point: To the middle of the forearm

Points to consider

Technique
- ☑ *Always* include both joints on the radiograph
- ☑ Lateral 1 – Flexed elbow
- ☑ Lateral 2 – full extension of the forearm and elbow
- ☑ Acute injury – horizontal beam *will* be necessary

kV	mAs	focus	film/screen	bucky	dose

Radiological assessment

☑ AP – slight superimposition of radial head over proximal ulna

☑ Lateral 2 – *Good* for bone alignment – radius and ulna superimposed

☒ *But* Lateral 2 – poor projection of the elbow – oblique elbow

☑ Lateral 1 – *Good* projection of the elbow and wrist joints

☒ Lateral 1 – Radius and ulna superimposed at the wrist, but separated at elbow

AP

- Patient seated, affected side towards the X-ray table
- Wrist, elbow and shoulder should be at the same level
- Forearm is fully supinated and rotated from the shoulder joint so that the hand and elbow are in a true AP position

Collimation

To include: PROXIMALLY: The elbow joint
DISTALLY: The wrist joint
LATERALLY: Soft tissue borders
MEDIALLY: Soft tissue borders

Lateral

- Elbow is flexed to 90°
- Wrist, elbow and shoulder should be at the same level
- Hand is rotated so that the styloid processes are superimposed

Collimation

To include: PROXIMALLY: The elbow joint
DISTALLY: The wrist joint
LATERALLY: Soft tissue borders
MEDIALLY: Soft tissue borders

ELBOW

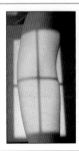 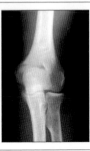

Projection: AP
Centring Point: 2.5 cm distal to a line joining the epicondyles

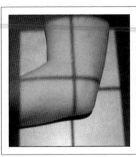 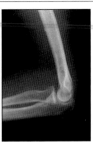

Projection: LATERAL
Centring Point: To the lateral epicondyle

Points to consider

Technique

- ☑ AP – epicondyles equidistant from the cassette
- ☑ AP – hand should be fully supinated
- ☑ Lateral – raise and immobilise the wrist on non-opaque pad; alternatively ask the patient to support the wrist with their opposite hand placed beneath the wrist of the affected limb
- ☑ Children – both elbows may be required for ossification centres
- ☒ Shoulder higher than the elbow is poor technique
- ☒ Possible supracondylar # – *never* forcibly extend the elbow

kV	mAs	focus	film/screen	bucky	dose

Radiological assessment

- ☑ Look for displaced fat pads – indication of trauma
- ☑ Common site of injury is the radial head
- ☑ Normally only the anterior distal fat pad is visible
- ☑ Check the elbow for avulsion #s – usually the result of a fall onto an outstretched hand
- ☑ Check soft tissue for swelling – a positive sign of trauma
- ☑ Supracondylar #s account for 60% of childhood #s

AP

- Patient seated, affected side towards the X-ray table
- Arm is fully supinated so that the epicondyles are equidistant from the cassette
- Wrist, elbow and shoulder should be at the same level

Collimation

To include: PROXIMALLY: The distal humerus
DISTALLY: The proximal radius and ulnar
LATERALLY: Soft tissue borders
MEDIALLY: Soft tissue borders

Lateral

- Elbow is flexed 90°
- Wrist, elbow and shoulder should be at the same level
- Hand is rotated so that the radial and ulnar styloid processes are superimposed

Collimation

To include: PROXIMALLY: The distal humerus
DISTALLY: The proximal radius and ulnar
LATERALLY: Soft tissue borders
MEDIALLY: Soft tissue borders

ELBOW

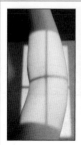 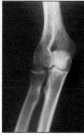

Projection: MODIFIED PROJECTIONS
1. POSSIBLE INJURY TO RADIAL HEAD

Centring Point: To the middle at the crease of the elbow

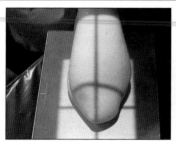 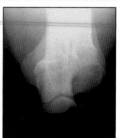

Projection: MODIFIED PROJECTIONS 2. FULL FLEXION OF THE ELBOW
Centring Point: 5 cm above the olecranon process

Points to consider

Technique

☑ 1. Use as a general projection in the case of severe trauma
☒ Difficult position to maintain – immobilisation essential

☑ 2. Ensure epicondyles are equidistant from the cassette
☑ Adjust the table to just below the shoulder level

kV	mAs	focus	film/screen	bucky	dose

Radiological assessment

☑ A visible fat pad is abnormal – probable #

☒ Radial head will be slightly superimposed on distal humerus

☑ Forearm and humerus should be superimposed

☑ Olecranon and distal humerus should be clearly seen

1. Possible injury to the radial head – general projection of the elbow joint

- Olecranon of the elbow is placed directly onto the cassette
- Patient leans slightly back so that both forearm and humerus form an angle of 45° to the cassette
- Sandbags may be employed to support the limbs

Collimation

To include: PROXIMALLY: Distal humerus
DISTALLY: Proximal radius and ulna
LATERALLY: Soft tissue borders
MEDIALLY: Soft tissue borders

2. Full flexion of the elbow

- Posterior aspect of the humerus is in contact with the cassette
- Hand placed onto the shoulder
- Epicondyles equidistant to the cassette

Collimation

To include: PROXIMALLY: Distal humerus and radius/ulna
DISTALLY: Olecranon process
LATERALLY: Soft tissue borders
MEDIALLY: Soft tissue borders

RADIAL HEAD

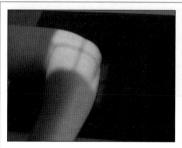 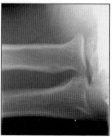

Projection: ALTERNATIVE PROJECTION

Centring Point: To the radial head. Central ray 45° to the humerus

Points to consider

Technique
- ☑ Ideally, hand is rotated with the thumb pointing upwards
- ☑ Painful joint – pronate the hand
- ☑ Take projection after the lateral – minimises movement
- ☑ Lead protection *must* be given – consider central ray
- ☒ Do not forcibly supinate hand

Radiological assessment
- ☑ Common injury due to a fall on an outstretched hand
- ☑ Radial head should be projected clear of the ulna
- ☑ Impacted head – slight angulation of the cortex of the neck
- ☑ Is there a positive fat pad sign?
- ☒ Image will be magnified and elongated

Alternative projection

- ● Patient seated with the affected arm placed upon the cassette
- ● Elbow is positioned as for the routine lateral projection

kV	mAs	focus	film/screen	bucky	dose

- Elbow is flexed to 90°
- Wrist and shoulder at the same level
- Wrist in true lateral position
- Central ray is angled *caudally* 45° to the forearm along the humeral axis

Collimation

To include: PROXIMALLY: Lower humerus and soft tissues
DISTALLY: Posterior elbow joint
LATERALLY: Soft tissue borders

HUMERUS

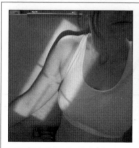 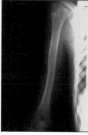

Projection: AP

Centring Point: To the middle of the humerus

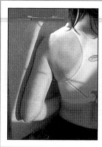 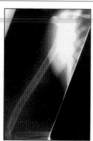

Projection: LATERAL

Centring Point: To the middle of the humerus

Points to consider

Technique

☑ Humerus should be abducted away from the trunk

☑ AP – elbow epicondyles equidistant from the cassette

☑ Lateral – hand, where possible, should be placed on abdomen

☑ *Must* include shoulder and elbow joints on the radiograph

☒ Acute injury – *do not* remove the arm from the sling

☒ Beware – breast shadows may obscure the humeral shaft

kV	mAs	focus	film/screen	bucky	dose

Radiological assessment

☑ #s occur at all levels – direct or indirect violence
☑ AP – head and greater tuberosity of humerus seen in profile
☑ Lateral – are the epicondyles superimposed?
☑ Common site in children – solitary bone cyst
☑ Adults – metastatic deposits – breast or bronchus
☒ Lateral – head of humerus *not* seen well – shoulder projection may be required

AP

● Patient may be supine or erect
● Body is rotated slightly onto the affected side so that the arm is in contact with the cassette
● Arm is fully supinated and slightly abducted where safe to do so
● Elbow epicondyles should be equidistant from the cassette

Lateral

● Patient may be prone or erect
● Body is rotated slightly onto the affected side so that the arm is in contact with the cassette – where possible and safe to do so the humerus is positioned completely clear of the thoracic wall
● Affected arm is carefully flexed and the hand is placed upon the upper abdomen
● Opposite arm is placed down by the side or the elbow flexed and hand used to support the hand/forearm of the injured side

Collimation

To include: PROXIMALLY: Shoulder joint
DISTALLY: Elbow joint
LATERALLY: Soft tissue borders
MEDIALLY: Soft tissue borders

2

Shoulder Girdle

SHOULDER JOINT

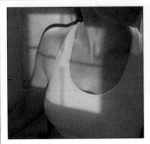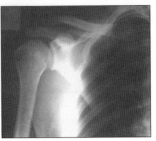

Projection: AP SHOULDER GIRDLE
Centring Point: 2.5 cm below the coracoid process

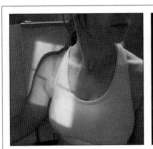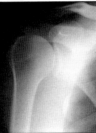

Projection: AP SHOULDER JOINT
Centring Point: To the coracoid process

Points to consider

Technique

- ☑ An axial projection of the shoulder may be required
- ☑ Exposure on *arrested* respiration
- ☒ *Never* forcibly abduct the humerus
- ☒ #ed clavicle – *do not* rotate patient – foreshortens the clavicle
- ☒ Lateral transthoracic – *do not* attempt because it increases radiation dose

kV	mAs	focus	film/screen	bucky	dose

Radiological assessment

☑ Anterior dislocation – humeral head below coracoid process
☑ Posterior dislocation – rare (about 5% of cases) – often overlooked, remember 'light bulb sign'
☑ Common site of # – surgical neck of humerus
☑ Check for impaction – # may be overlooked
☑ Acute inflammation – look for calcification – rotator cuff muscles

AP shoulder girdle

This projection gives a general assessment of the shoulder girdle

● Patient may be supine or erect facing the X-ray tube
● Body is very slightly rotated onto the affected side
● Arm is abducted from the body and supinated

Collimation

To include: SUPERIORLY: Clavicle
INFERIORLY: Inferior angle of the scapula
LATERALLY: Soft tissues
MEDIALLY: Sternoclavicular joint

AP shoulder joint

● Patient may be supine or erect facing the X-ray table
● Body rotated approximately 40° to the affected side so that the scapula is parallel to the cassette
● If possible, arm partially abducted and supinated

Collimation

To include: SUPERIORLY: Clavicle
INFERIORLY: Proximal third of humerus
LATERALLY: Soft tissues
MEDIALLY: Lateral third of clavicle

SHOULDER JOINT

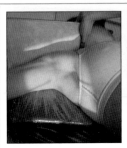 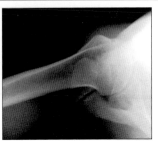

Projection: AXIAL INFEROSUPERIOR

Centring Point: To the axilla – small angulation to the joint

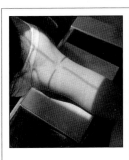 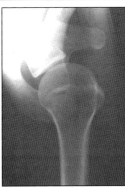

Projection: AXIAL SUPEROINFERIOR

Centring Point: To the acromion process with 10° angulation away from the body

Points to consider

Technique

☑ Superoinferior – only use when full abduction is possible

☑ *Must* include the glenohumeral joint on the radiograph

☑ Inferosuperior – when only limited abduction possible

kV	mAs	focus	film/screen	bucky	dose

☑ Axial projection should be taken in all cases of trauma

☒ Acute injury – *never* forcibly abduct the arm

☑ Consider the alternative 'Y' projection

Radiological assessment

☑ Glenoid seen between coracoid, glenoid and acromion processes

☑ #s of coracoid and infraspinous processes can be clearly seen

☑ Children – epiphyseal lines vary – not to be confused with #s

☑ Check soft tissues for calcification of rotator cuff muscles

☒ Bicipital groove should not be confused with a #

Axial inferosuperior

- Patient supine on the X-ray table
- Ideally the affected arm is abducted to 90°
- Hand turned with palm facing upwards
- Cassette supported vertically against the shoulder and gently pressed into the neck with patient's head turned away from beam
- Place a non-opaque pad under the affected shoulder to ensure that the cassette's lower margin can be placed lower than the area of interest

Collimation

To include: ANTERIORLY: Anterior soft tissues
POSTERIORLY: Posterior soft tissues
DISTALLY: Upper humerus
PROXIMALLY: Glenohumeral joint

Axial superoinferior

- Patient seated at the side of the X-ray table
- Body is inclined towards the table, head turned away from beam
- Affected arm is abducted as much as possible over a cassette
- Elbow rests upon the table top
- Palm of the hand is facing downwards

Collimation

To include: ANTERIORLY: Anterior soft tissues
POSTERIORLY: Posterior soft tissues
DISTALLY: Upper humerus
PROXIMALLY: Glenohumeral joint

SHOULDER JOINT

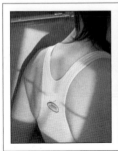 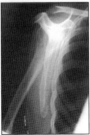

Projection: SUPPLEMENTARY 'Y' PROJECTION

Centring Point: Just medial to the midpoint of the palpable scapula. Horizontal central ray

Points to consider

Technique

- ☑ Projection useful in the evaluation of possible shoulder dislocation
- ☑ Visualise upper humeral head and lateral scapula
- ☑ Position of the arm is not critical, but should be placed for comfort
- ☑ Exposure on arrested respiration

Radiological assessment

- ☑ Y is formed by acromion, coracoid and lateral border of scapula
- ☑ Normally head of humerus should sit at junction of the Y
- ☑ Anterior dislocation – humeral head beneath coracoid process
- ☑ Posterior dislocation – humeral head beneath acromion process
- ☒ Scapula should not be superimposed over the rib cage

Supplementary 'Y' projection – dislocated shoulder

- Patient is in the erect position and facing the cassette in the upright stand
- Arm nearest the bucky is relaxed and the back of the hand placed on the hip
- Opposite arm holds onto the erect bucky for support
- Trunk is rotated approximately 60° away from the side under examination
- Anterior surface of the shoulder under examination is in contact with the cassette

kV	mAs	focus	film/screen	bucky	dose

Collimation

To include: SUPERIORLY: Clavicle
INFERIORLY: Scapulae and proximal humerus
LATERALLY: Humerus
MEDIALLY: Scapulae and rib cage

AP apical oblique

● Patient is positioned as for an AP shoulder joint

● Body is rotated 40°/45° to the affected side

● Centre to the coracoid process with 45° caudal angulation

Due to the angulation there is distortion of the image but soft tissue changes not visible on a routine AP shoulder joint and the position of the humeral head can be seen.

SCAPULA

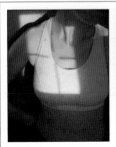 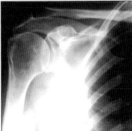

Projection: AP

Centring Point: 8 cm below the midpoint of the clavicle

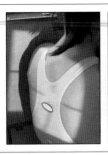 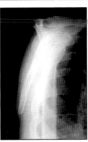

Projection: LATERAL

Centring Point: Just medial to the midpoint of the palpable scapula. Horizontal central ray

Points to consider

Technique

- ✓ AP – better images are obtained if you use a bucky
- ✓ Exposure on *arrrested* expiration
- ✗ *Never* forcibly abduct the humerus
- ✗ Lateral – failure to abduct the arm results in humerus superimposed on the scapula

kV	mAs	focus	film/screen	bucky	dose

Radiological assessment

☑ AP – the whole of the scapula *must* be included

☑ #s – usually the result of a direct crush-type injury

☑ Lateral – scapula blade *must* be clear of the rib cage

☒ Humerus should not superimpose the region of interest

AP

- Patient may be supine or erect facing the X-ray tube – erect preferred to avoid pressure on scapula
- Body is very slightly rotated onto the affected side by approximately 30°
- Arm is abducted from the body and supinated

Collimation

To include: SUPERIORLY: Clavicle
               INFERIORLY: Inferior angle of the scapula
               LATERALLY: Soft tissues
               MEDIALLY: Sternoclavicular joint

Lateral

- Patient may be prone or erect facing the bucky with the affected shoulder in close contact
- Trunk is rotated so that the blade of the scapula is perpendicular to the bucky
- Affected arm is abducted away from the body

Collimation

To include: SUPERIORLY: Acromioclavicular joint
               INFERIORLY: Inferior angle of the scapula
               LATERALLY: Soft tissue borders
               MEDIALLY: Lateral rib cage

ACROMIOCLAVICULAR JOINTS

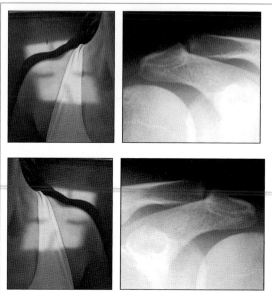

Projection: AP AND AP WEIGHT-BEARING

Centring Point: To the palpable acromioclavicular joint. Horizontal central ray

Points to consider

Technique

☑ Two exposures – centre to each acromioclavicular joint in turn

☑ Exposure on arrested respiration

☑ Repeat examination with patient holding weights

☑ Patient must hold weights in both hands for at least 3 min before examination – allows gravity effect to take place

☒ *Do not* use one exposure with open collimation for both joints on one radiograph – consider dose to thyroid

kV	mAs	focus	film/screen	bucky	dose

Radiological assessment

- ☑ Both radiographs should be comparable
- ☑ Normal size of joint space less than 10 mm in adult
- ☑ Clearly identify which are the weight-bearing radiographs
- ☑ Possible subluxation – clavicle will lift and separate from the acromion due to a tear in the acromioclavicular joint capsule
- ☒ Assessment line – normally inferior aspect of the acromion and clavicle should be in a straight line

AP and AP weight-bearing

- Patient erect facing the X-ray tube
- Arms are placed down by the side of the trunk and are relaxed
- Posterior aspect of the shoulder under examination is in contact with the cassette
- Patient's trunk is rotated approximately 10° to the side under examination
- Both acromioclavicular joints may be required for comparison

Collimation

Precise collimation to include the acromioclavicular joint

CLAVICLE

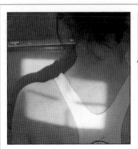
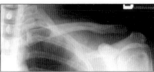

Projection: PA

Centring Point: To the centre of the clavicle. Horizontal central ray

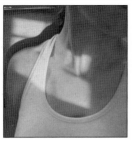
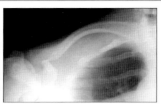

Projection: INFEROSUPERIOR

Centring Point: To the centre of the clavicle. Central ray 20° cephalad

Points to consider

Technique

☑ PA – increased definition is due to decreased object film distance

☑ Exposure on *arrested* respiration

☑ Inferosuperior – ensure the clavicle is not projected off the cassette

kV	mAs	focus	film/screen	bucky	dose

Radiological assessment

- ☑ Clavicle #s are often comminuted and easy to detect
- ☑ Majority of #s involve the middle third
- ☑ *Must* include the medial end of the clavicle
- ☑ Inferosuperior – clavicle should be demonstrated clear of any superimposed shadows

PA

- Patient can be prone or erect facing the cassette
- Affected shoulder is rotated slightly to bring the clavicle in close contact with the cassette
- Patient's head is rotated away from the side being examined
- Arms are placed down by the patient's side

Collimation

To include the whole of the clavicle

Inferosuperior

- Patient can be supine or erect facing the X-ray tube
- Patient's shoulder is in close contact with the cassette
- Patient's head is rotated away from the side being examined
- Arms are placed down by the patient's side
- Cassette is displaced superiorly

Collimation

To include the whole of the clavicle

3

Thoracic Cage

UPPER RIBS

- Right or left posterior obliques — 48
- Lower ribs – AP — 48

STERNUM

- Lateral — 50
- Anterior oblique (RAO) — 50

UPPER RIBS

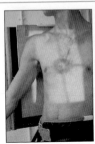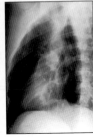

Projection: RIGHT OR LEFT POSTERIOR OBLIQUES

Centring Point: In the mid-clavicular line of the side under examination – at level of the midpoint of the sternal body. Horizontal central ray

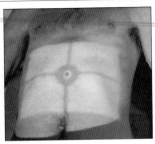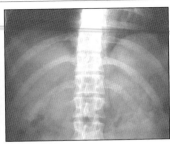

Projection: LOWER RIBS – AP

Centring Point: To a point in the midline midway between the xiphisternum and the lower costal margin

Points to consider

Technique

- ☒ Trauma – oblique ribs not always necessary – rarely changes management of the patient
- ☑ Oblique – exposure on arrested full inspiration
- ☑ Oblique – patient erect – better with inspiration
- ☑ AP – exposure on arrested expiration to show the maximum number of ribs below the diaphragm

kV	mAs	focus	film/screen	bucky	dose

Radiological assessment

☑ Check each rib for # – it is rare to see displacement due to the numerous attached muscles

☒ Oblique – ribs away from cassette will be foreshortened

☑ Oblique – posterior rib articulations seen well on the raised side

☑ #s of ribs will unite spontaneously – treatment is limited

☑ Look for metastatic deposits – associated with rib destruction

Right or left posterior obliques

- Patient supine or erect, facing the X-ray tube
- Body rotated approximately 45° onto the affected side
- Arms are abducted away from the trunk

Collimation

To include: SUPERIORLY: First rib
INFERIORLY: Diaphragms
LATERALLY: Rib cage

Lower ribs – AP

- Patient lies supine on the X-ray table
- Shoulders and anterior superior iliac spines (ASIS) equidistant from the table top

Collimation

To include: SUPERIORLY: Diaphragms
INFERIORLY: Lower costal margin
LATERALLY: Rib cage and abdominal wall

STERNUM

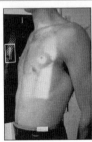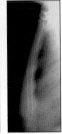

Projection: LATERAL

Centring Point: To a point 3 cm below the sternal angle. Horizontal central ray. SID 150 cm

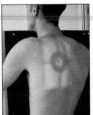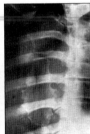

Projection: ANTERIOR OBLIQUE (RAO)

Centring Point: To a point 8 cm lateral to the palpable fifth thoracic vertebra on the side furthest from the cassette. Horizontal central ray

Points to consider

Technique

☑ A grid or bucky is essential for both projections

☑ Lateral – exposure on arrested full inspiration

☑ Lateral – greater SID of 150 cm will decrease magnification

☑ Oblique – patient allowed to breathe gently during exposure

☑ Right anterior oblique – cardiac shadow will help visualise the sternum

kV	mAs	focus	film/screen	bucky	dose

Radiological assessment

☑ *Must* include from the sternoclavicular joint to xiphisternum

☒ Sternum *must not* be overpenetrated

☑ Gentle breathing will blur the rib shadows

☒ Obliquity – the spine and sternum *must not* be superimposed

☒ Over-rotation – sternum outside cardiac shadow

Lateral

● Patient erect

● Median sagittal plane is parallel to the erect bucky

● Patient's shoulders are rotated posteriorly

● Arms placed behind the trunk and shoulders and gently pulled back

Collimation

To include: SUPERIORLY: Acromioclavicular joints
INFERIORLY: Xiphisternum
ANTERIORLY: Anterior soft tissues
POSTERIORLY: Posterior sternum

Anterior oblique (RAO)

● Patient erect facing the cassette

● Trunk is rotated approximately 30° so that the right side of the body is in contact with the erect bucky

● Arms are placed around the erect bucky to maintain stability

Collimation

To include: SUPERIORLY: Acromioclavicular joints
INFERIORLY: Xiphisternum
LATERALLY: Costal cartilage

4

Respiratory System

LUNG FIELDS

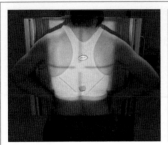
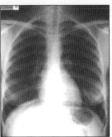

Projection: PA

Centring Point: To the palpable sixth thoracic vertebra. Horizontal central ray angled 5° caudad. SID 180 cm

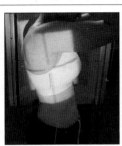
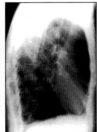

Projection: LATERAL

Centring Point: Mid-axillary line at the level sixth thoracic vertebra. Horizontal central ray. SID 180 cm

Points to consider

Technique

☑ PA – radiograph *must* be taken on full inspiration

☑ PA – possible pneumothorax – radiograph taken on full expiration

☑ Make sure the scapulae are clear of the lung fields

☒ If the patient cannot place their hands on hips – turn the hands internally and place the arms around the cassette

☒ Reminder to remove jewellery – necklaces

kV	mAs	focus	film/screen	bucky	dose

Radiological assessment

☑ Poor inspiration may mimic cardiac enlargement

☑ Small pneumothorax best seen on an expiration radiograph

☑ Full inspiration – right 8–9 posterior ribs are just clear of the diaphragm

☑ Haemoptysis – look for evidence of lung cancer or tuberculosis

☑ Breathlessness – look for heart failure or collapse of lobes

PA

● Patient facing the cassette with chin extended

● Trunk is adjusted so that the median sagittal plane is perpendicular to the cassette

● Feet are parted to maintain stability

● Dorsal aspect of the hands are placed behind and below the hips and the elbows are brought forwards

● Shoulders are relaxed and rotated forwards until they are in contact with the cassette

● Instruct patient *not* to raise their shoulders as they breathe in

Collimation

To include: SUPERIORLY: Apices
             INFERIORLY: Costophrenic angles
             LATERALLY: Soft tissue borders

Lateral

● Patient is rotated to bring the lung under examination in contact with the cassette

● Median sagittal plane is parallel to the cassette

● Patient's arms are folded over the head or can be raised to rest on a suitable support

Collimation

To include: SUPERIORLY: Apices
             INFERIORLY: Costophrenic angles
             ANTERIORLY: Sternum and anterior ribs
             POSTERIORLY: Posterior rib cage

LUNG FIELDS

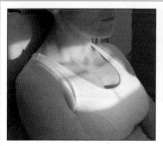
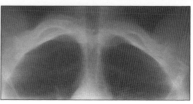

Projection: APICES
Centring Point: To the sternal angle. Horizontal central ray

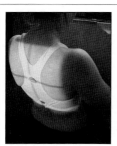
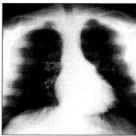

Projection: LORDOTIC
Centring Point: To the palpable sixth thoracic vertebra. Horizontal central ray

Points to consider

Technique

☑ Apices – use if an opacity is obscured by ribs or clavicular shadows

☑ Apices – ensure both shoulders are level and touching the cassette

☑ Apices – if patient cannot lean back angle the tube 30° cephalad

☑ Both projections – exposure on arrested inspiration

☑ Lordotic – to demonstrate a right middle lobe collapse or an interlobar pleural effusion

kV	mAs	focus	film/screen	bucky	dose

Radiological assessment

☑ Clavicles *must* be projected clear of the apices

☒ Apices – if clavicles are superimposed upon lung fields there is not enough angulation

☑ Lordotic – the middle lobe fissure should be horizontal

☑ Haemoptysis – look for evidence of lung cancer or tuberculosis

☑ Check the heart outline – an ill-defined right heart border may be the result of a middle lobe consolidation

Apices

● Patient seated and facing the X-ray tube with their back a short distance from the cassette

● Trunk is then carefully reclined so that the coronal plane is approximately 30–40° to the cassette

Collimation

To include: SUPERIORLY: Apices
INFERIORLY: Upper lung fields
LATERALLY: Rib cage

Lordotic

● Patient is positioned as for a routine PA chest examination

● Hands securely clasp the erect bucky or cassette stand

● Patient leans backwards towards the X-ray tube by approximately 30–40°

Collimation

To include: SUPERIORLY: Apices
INFERIORLY: Diaphragms
LATERALLY: Rib cage

TRACHEA–THORACIC INLET

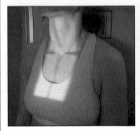 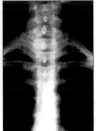

Projection: AP
Centring Point: To the sternal notch. Horizontal central ray

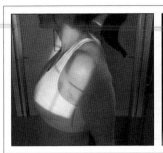 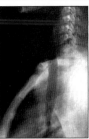

Projection: LATERAL
Centring Point: Just posterior to the sternal notch. Horizontal central ray. SID 150 cm

Points to consider

Technique

☑ AP – patient can be erect or supine, but supine results in greater immobilisation

☑ Lateral – patient can be standing or seated

☑ Lateral – if patient standing, weight *must* be equally distributed

☑ Exposure while patient employs Valsalva manoeuvre

kV	mAs	focus	film/screen	bucky	dose

Radiological assessment

☑ AP – *must* include from mid-cervical to mid-thoracic region

☑ Lateral – *must* include from mid-cervical to mid-thoracic region

☒ Shoulders *must* not superimpose the trachea

☑ AP and lateral – trachea should be demonstrated when filled with air

AP

- Patient supine on the X-ray table
- Shoulders equidistant from the table top
- Median sagittal plane perpendicular
- Chin is raised slightly

Collimation

To include: SUPERIORLY: Body of fourth cervical vertebra
INFERIORLY: Bifurcation of trachea/carina (5th/6th thoracic vertebra)
LATERALLY: The spinous processes

Lateral

- Patient erect with a shoulder in contact with the erect bucky
- Median sagittal plane is parallel to the bucky
- Arms are placed behind the trunk and the hands clasped together
- Shoulders are rotated posteriorly as far as possible to bring the thorax forwards

Collimation

To include: ANTERIORLY: Manubrium of sternum
POSTERIORLY: Thoracic spine
SUPERIORLY: Body of fourth cervical vertebra
INFERIORLY: Bifurcation of trachea (fourth thoracic vertebra)

5

Abdominal Contents

ABDOMEN

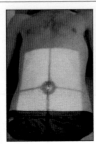 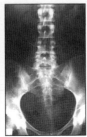

Projection: AP SUPINE

Centring Point: In the midline at the level of iliac crests

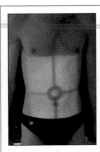 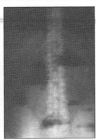

Projection: AP ERECT

Centring Point: In the midline at the level of lower costal margin. Horizontal central ray

Points to consider

Technique

- ☑ Acute abdomen – *must* include an *erect* chest radiograph
- ☑ Exposure – usually on arrested expiration
- ☑ Place pads under the knees to aid comfort for the patient
- ☑ Use gonad protection for male patients
- ☒ Erect abdomen – adds little diagnostic information – possibly use other modalities – possibly ultrasound first, then consider CT

kV	mAs	focus	film/screen	bucky	dose

Radiological assessment

☑ Check the size of organs – a knowledge of anatomy is essential

☑ Symphysis pubis *must* be included on the radiograph

☑ Pneumoperitoneum – commonest cause is a perforated peptic ulcer

☑ Normal small bowel gas pattern should *not* exceed 2.5 cm

☑ Acute abdomen – check lower ribs and lumbar transverse processes if #s present – consider injury to liver, spleen or kidney

☑ Check fat and soft tissue interfaces – not always visible, but loss of markings can be an indication of pathology

AP supine

● Patient lies supine upon the X-ray table

● Median sagittal plane is perpendicular and the anterior superior iliac spines (ASIS) are equidistant to the table top

● A pad may be placed under the knees for support

● Ensure patients hands are by their side and not under the pelvis

Collimation

To include: SUPERIORLY: Diaphragm
 INFERIORLY: Symphysis pubis
 LATERALLY: Soft tissue borders

AP erect

● Patient is erect with the back leaning against the upright bucky

● Median sagittal plane is perpendicular and the ASIS are equidistant to the erect bucky

● Immobilisation bands can be applied to support the patient in this position

Collimation

To include: SUPERIORLY: Diaphragm
 INFERIORLY: ASIS
 LATERALLY: Soft tissue borders

ABDOMEN

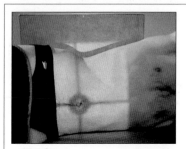

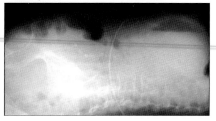

Projection: LEFT LATERAL DECUBITUS

Centring Point: In the midline at the level of iliac crests. Horizontal central ray

Points to consider

Technique

- ☑ Useful alternative to the erect if the patient is immobile
- ☑ Acute abdomen – position patient for at least 5 min before making an exposure – enables free gas to rise and redistribute
- ☑ Vertical gridded cassette – position as close to abdomen as possible
- ☑ *Right* marker on upper cassette – anatomically correct

Radiological assessment

- ☑ Will demonstrate the whole of left hemidiaphragm and part of right hemidiaphragm – free gas will collect at this point

kV	mAs	focus	film/screen	bucky	dose

☑ Exposure should demonstrate soft tissue of abdominal wall

☑ Remember chest radiograph – chest disease can mimic an acute abdomen

☒ Overpenetration for bony anatomy is less important

Left lateral decubitus

● Patient lies on the left side

● Elbows and arms are flexed and placed by the side of the head

● Median sagittal plane is parallel to the table top

● Hips and knees are slightly flexed to maintain stability

Collimation

To include: SUPERIORLY: Diaphragm
INFERIORLY: ASIS
LATERALLY: Lateral abdominal walls
(contrast studies *must* include the rectum)

URINARY TRACT

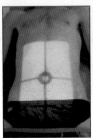 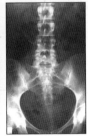

Projection: AP SUPINE – KIDNEY, URETER AND BLADDER (KUB)

Centring Point: In the midline at level of iliac crests and adjusted to include the symphysis pubis on the cassette

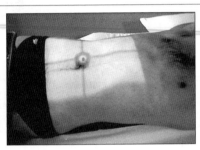 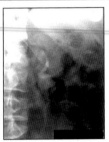

Projection: KIDNEY/URETER POSTERIOR OBLIQUES

Centring Point: In the mid-clavicular line – on the raised side at the level of the lower costal margin

Points to consider

Technique

☑ AP – the symphysis pubis *must* be included on the radiograph

☑ AP – exposure in full inspiration is so all urinary tract is visualised. Position of kidneys alters during respiration, higher in abdomen in expiration

☑ Use gonad protection for male patients

☑ Renal colic – a limited IVU is highly accurate in confirming the diagnosis

kV	mAs	focus	film/screen	bucky	dose

Radiological assessment

☑ Check that the upper poles of the kidneys are included

☒ *Do not* confuse renal stones and pelvic phleboliths

☑ Approximately 85% of renal stones are radiopaque

☑ Pelvic phleboliths have a round radiopaque halo surrounding a small lucent centre

☑ Oblique – kidney closer to the cassette seen in profile, kidney away from the cassette seen *en face*

AP supine – KUB

● Patient lies supine upon the X-ray table

● Median sagittal plane is perpendicular and the ASIS are equidistant to the table top

● A pad may be placed under the knees for support

Collimation

To include: SUPERIORLY: Upper pole of kidney
INFERIORLY: Symphysis pubis
LATERALLY: Both kidneys

Kidney/ureter posterior obliques

● Patient lies supine upon the X-ray table

● Unaffected side of the trunk is raised approximately 20–30° and supported in this position with non-opaque pads

● Arms and elbows are flexed and placed at the side of the head

● Hips and knees are slightly flexed to maintain stability

Collimation

To include: Precise collimation to include both or a specific kidney

URINARY TRACT

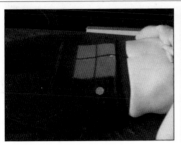 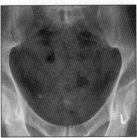

Projection: AP BLADDER

Centring Point: In the midline 5 cm above the symphysis pubis

Central ray 15° caudad

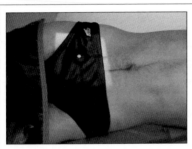 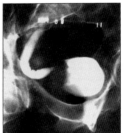

Projection: BLADDER POSTERIOR OBLIQUES

Centring Point: 2.5 cm above the symphysis pubis

Points to consider

Technique

☑ Symphysis pubis *must* be included on the radiograph

☑ Lower bowel preparation is an advantage

☑ Gonad protection for the male patient

☑ Raise affected side to demonstrate insertion of ureter into the bladder

kV	mAs	focus	film/screen	bucky	dose

Radiological assessment

☑ Contrast media – will identify bladder retention or prolapse

☑ Oblique – will differentiate between calculus in the bladder and calculi outside the bladder

☑ Radiograph above contains contrast media to appreciate the size and position of the bladder

AP bladder

- Patient lies supine upon the X-ray table
- Median sagittal plane is perpendicular and the ASIS are equidistant to the table top
- A pad may be placed under the knees for support

Collimation

To include: SUPERIORLY: Sacrum
INFERIORLY: Symphysis pubis
LATERALLY: Pelvic brim

Bladder posterior obliques

- Patient lies supine upon the X-ray table
- Affected side of the trunk is raised approximately 30–40° and supported in this position with non-opaque pads
- Arms and elbows are flexed and placed at the side of the head
- Hips and knees are slightly flexed to maintain stability

Collimation

To include: SUPERIORLY: Sacrum
INFERIORLY: Symphysis pubis
LATERALLY: Pelvic brim

6 Pelvis, Hip Joint and Upper Third of Femur

PELVIS

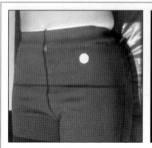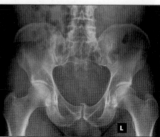

Projection: AP

Centring Point: Midline midway between the ASIS and the superior border of the symphysis pubis (photograph – solid while circle denotes ASIS)

Points to consider

Technique

- ☑ Rotate the legs approximately 15° medially and support
- ☑ Large patient – raise the SID to 120 cm to reduce magnification, but care with exposure and dose
- ☒ Exposure – too high a mAs will blacken out the iliac fossa
- ☒ *Do not* place arms by side – they may appear on the radiograph

Radiological assessment

- ☒ Foreshortened femoral neck – inadequate medial rotation
- ☑ Check obturator foramina are equal size and shape
- ☑ Whole of the pelvis *must* be included on the radiograph
- ☑ Check Shenton's line – any disruption is due to a fractured neck of femur
- ☒ *Do not* confuse epiphyseal lines with #s – iliac crest fuses late teens to early twenties

kV	mAs	focus	film/screen	bucky	dose

Note

Obliques of the pelvis may be required to demonstrate:

- On the raised side – iliac crest in profile and into the acetabular fossa
- On the non-raised side – iliac fossa opened out and the acetabulum in profile

AP

- Patient lies supine in the centre of the table
- ASIS must be equidistant from the table top
- Both knees are *very* slightly flexed and supported by non-opaque pads
- Heels are separated and the limbs are rotated internally until the toes are touching. NB Should not be forced in a trauma situation

Collimation

To include: SUPERIORLY: Body of fifth lumbar vertebra and iliac crests
             INFERIORLY: Proximal femurs
             LATERALLY: Soft tissue borders

BOTH HIPS

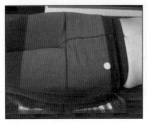 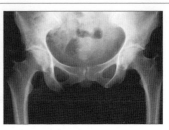

Projection: AP

Centring Point: Midline 2.5 cm superior to the symphysis pubis (photograph – solid while circle denotes ASIS)

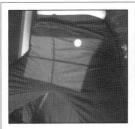 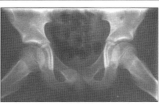

Projection: LATERAL (FROG)

Centring Point: Midline 2.5 cm superior to the symphysis pubis (photograph – solid while circle denotes ASIS)

Points to consider

Technique

☑ Both hips and femur should be symmetrical

☑ Trauma – *no* gonad protection is needed for first examination *only*

☑ Keep the hands away from the pelvis

☑ Place a small pad under the knees to ensure patient comfort

kV	mAs	focus	film/screen	bucky	dose

☒ *Do not* forcibly rotate the limb if possible fractured neck of femur

☑ Whole length of a prosthesis and its cement should be included

Radiological assessment

☑ AP – allows comparison between both hips

☑ Femoral epiphysis present from 3 months to 18–20 years

☑ Break in cortical outline or interruption in cortical pattern – #

☑ Perthes' disease – more common in boys and rare over 7 years of age

☑ Slipped epiphysis – more common in boys and rare under 8 years of age

AP

- Patient lies supine
- Anterior superior iliac spines (ASIS) are equidistant from the table top
- Heels are separated and the limbs rotated medially approximately 10° and supported by sandbags

Collimation

To include: SUPERIORLY: ASIS
INFERIORLY: Upper third of femur
LATERALLY: Ilium and soft tissues

Lateral (frog)

- Patient lies supine
- ASIS are equidistant from the table top
- Hips and knees are flexed
- Knees are separated and rotated laterally approximately 60° so that the plantar aspects of the feet are in contact with each other
- Patient is supported with sandbags and non-opaque pads

Collimation

To include: SUPERIORLY: ASIS
INFERIORLY: Upper femur
LATERALLY: Ilium and soft tissues

SINGLE HIP

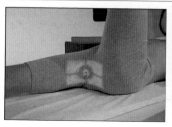 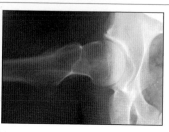

Projection: LATERAL – NECK OF FEMUR

Centring Point: So the central ray emerges at the level of the greater trochanter. Horizontal central ray perpendicular to the cassette

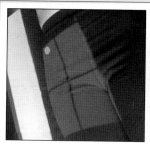 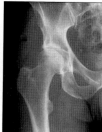

Projection: AP – SINGLE HIP

Centring Point: 2.5 cm distally along a perpendicular bisector of a line joining the ASIS and the symphysis pubis (photograph – solid while circle denotes ASIS)

Points to consider

Technique

- ☑ Lateral – ensure to maintain the SID
- ☑ Lateral – the opposite limb *must* be securely supported
- ☑ Lateral – ensure the central ray is not directed at the control panel or a door
- ☑ Lateral – horizontal beam *must* be perpendicular to cassette
- ☒ Trauma – *never* forcibly rotate the affected limb

kV	mAs	focus	film/screen	bucky	dose

Radiological assessment

- ☑ Look for any increased density – may be due to an impacted #
- ☑ Undisplaced fractured neck of femur – discontinuity in trabecular lines
- ☑ Complication of fractured neck of femur – avascular necrosis of femoral head
- ☑ Bright light may be required to view the image
- ☑ Positive # – a chest radiograph *will* be required

Lateral – neck of femur

- Patient lies supine with the affected leg extended
- Rotate the limb so that the foot is vertical – care *must* be taken not to exacerbate the injury
- Opposite limb is raised so that the femur is in a vertical position
- Opposite knee is flexed and supported
- Gridded stationary cassette is positioned vertically with one edge placed against the patient's waist
- Cassette is adjusted so that it is parallel to the neck of femur and is supported in position with a 45° pad

Collimation

Precise collimation by the use of a cone or diaphragm to include the acetabulum and neck of femur

AP – single hip

- Patient lies supine with the affected hip in the centre of the table
- Pelvis is adjusted so that the ASIS are equidistant from the table top
- Affected limb is rotated so that the foot is vertical and supported

Collimation

To include the whole of the hip joint

SINGLE HIP

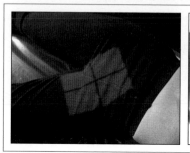 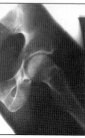

Projection:
LATERAL (NON-TRAUMA)

Centring Point:
Directly to the femoral head

Points to consider

Technique

☑ *Only* to be used when a # is not suspected
☑ Place a non-opaque pad under the knee for support
☑ Oblique the pelvis slightly to aid patient's comfort
☑ Care with exposure – especially if an automatic exposure device (AED) is used

Radiological assessment

☑ Neck of femur should appear in the centre of the radiograph
☑ Greater trochanter should be superimposed over the neck of femur
☑ Lesser trochanter is seen on the medial aspect
☒ Over-rotation – the obturator foramen appears closed

Lateral (non-trauma)

● Patient lies supine upon the X-ray table
● Joint under examination is adjusted so that it is central to the table
● Trunk is rotated approximately 45° onto the affected side
● Hip and knee of the side being examined are slightly flexed and the knee is in close contact with the table top

kV	mAs	focus	film/screen	bucky	dose

- Opposite limb is raised and supported in this position
- Long axis of collimation should follow the line of the femur

Collimation

To include: PROXIMALLY: ASIS
              DISTALLY: Upper shaft of femur
              LATERALLY: Soft tissue borders
              MEDIALLY: Obturator foramen

7 Lower Extremity

TOES

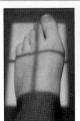 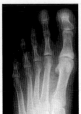 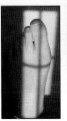 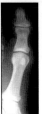

Projection: DORSIPLANTAR (AP)
Centring Point: To the third metatarsophalangeal joint

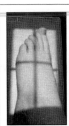 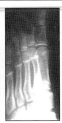

Projection: DORSIPLANTAR (AP OBLIQUE)
Centring Point: To the third metatarsophalangeal joint

Points to consider

Technique

☑ Always include the phalanges and distal metatarsals
☑ Care with exposure – overpenetration of distal phalanges
☑ Try using an aluminium filter for the optimal exposure
☑ For the great toe – centre to proximal interphalangeal joint

kV	mAs	focus	film/screen	bucky	dose

Radiological assessment

☑ Freiburg's infarction – osteochondritis of the second metatarsal head

☑ Osteomyelitis – soft tissue swelling and irregular depleted bone

☑ Trabeculae should be uniform or change gradually

☑ Extensive soft tissue swelling – severe injury or bone infection

☑ Phalanges and metatarsals of each toe should lie straight

Dorsiplantar (AP)

● Patient sitting with hips and knees flexed

● Affected foot is placed with the plantar aspect upon the cassette

Collimation

To include: PROXIMALLY: Metatarsals
　　　　　　DISTALLY: Phalanges
　　　　　　LATERALLY: Soft tissue borders
　　　　　　MEDIALLY: Soft tissue borders

Dorsiplantar (AP oblique)

● Patient sitting with hips and knees flexed

● Affected foot is placed with the plantar aspect upon the cassette

● Leg is medially rotated so that the foot is at an angle of approximately 30–40° to the cassette

● Non-opaque pad used if necessary

Collimation

To include: PROXIMALLY: Metatarsals
　　　　　　DISTALLY: Phalanges
　　　　　　LATERALLY: Soft tissue borders
　　　　　　MEDIALLY: Soft tissue borders

TOES

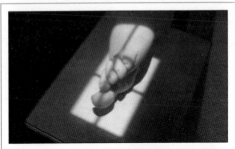

Projection: LATERAL

Centring Point: To the first metatarsophalangeal joint

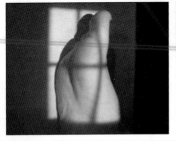 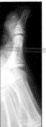

Points to consider

Technique

- ☒ True lateral – limited value as the toes are superimposed
- ☑ To isolate a specific toe – use a non-opaque pad
- ☒ *Do not* forcibly separate the toes – exacerbates injury
- ☑ Slightly flex the knee to aid positioning and comfort
- ☑ Try raising the cassette upon a pad before positioning

Radiological assessment

- ☑ Sesamoid bones of the great toe arise from two or more centres
- ☑ Failure to unite – may resemble an epiphyseal #

kV	mAs	focus	film/screen	bucky	dose

☑ Trabeculae should be uniform or change gradually

☒ Projection has limited value apart from assessing the extent of any displacement

Lateral

- Patient lies:
  - For the first, second and third toes – on the side opposite to that being examined
  - Medial side of the foot and leg under examination is placed in contact with the table top
  - For the fourth and fifth toes – on the side under examination
  - Lateral side of the foot and leg under examination is placed in contact with the table top
- Plantar aspect of the foot is at right angles to the cassette
- A pad is placed under the ankle to maintain the position

Collimation

To include: PROXIMALLY: Metatarsals
DISTALLY: Phalanges
LATERALLY: Soft tissue borders
MEDIALLY: Soft tissue borders

FOOT

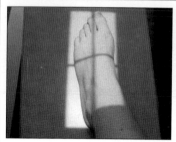 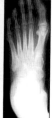

Projection: DORSIPLANTAR (AP)

Centring Point: To the cuboid–navicular joint, 10° cephalic angulation to demonstrate tarsal bones

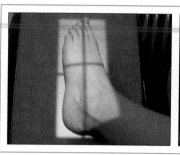 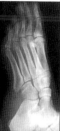

Projection: DORSIPLANTAR (AP OBLIQUE)

Centring Point: To the cuboid–navicular joint

Points to consider

Technique

- ☑ Slight angulation of tube towards the ankle – this will open the articulations of the foot
- ☑ Oblique – metatarsals free from superimposition
- ☑ Consider using a wedge filter for optimum penetration
- ☑ Ensure knee is flexed to prevent the cassette from slipping

kV	mAs	focus	film/screen	bucky	dose

Radiological assessment

☑ Lisfranc injury – # through base of second metatarsal and dislocation of third, fourth and fifth metatarsals

☑ Accessory ossification centre – base of fifth metatarsal – bone contours smooth and rounded with intact cortical margins

☑ Look for periosteal thickening – stress #

☑ Oblique – consider the anterior calcaneum for avulsion #s

Dorsiplantar (AP)

● Patient sitting with hips and knees flexed
● Affected foot is placed with the plantar aspect upon the cassette
● Leg can be supported by the opposite leg

Collimation

To include: PROXIMALLY: Head of talus
DISTALLY: Great toe
LATERALLY: Soft tissue borders
MEDIALLY: Soft tissue borders

Dorsiplantar (AP oblique)

● Patient sitting with hips and knees flexed
● Affected foot is placed with the plantar aspect upon the cassette
● Leg is medially rotated so that the foot is at an angle of approximately 30–40° to the cassette
● Non-opaque pad is placed under the foot

Collimation

To include: PROXIMALLY: Head of talus
DISTALLY: Great toe
LATERALLY: Soft tissue borders
MEDIALLY: Soft tissue borders

FOOT

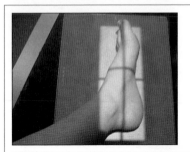

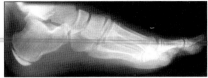

Projection: LATERAL

Centring Point: To the navicular–cuneiform joint

Points to consider

Technique

☑ This projection is used when a foreign body is suspected or an additional projection for # or dislocation

☑ Lateral projection *must* include the whole of calcaneum

☒ *Do not* overpenetrate the calcaneum

☑ Place a pad under the knee to maintain the position

Radiological assessment

☑ Check the alignment of the talonavicular and calcaneocuboid bones

☑ Look for breaks in the cortical bone or bony trabeculae

☑ Soft tissue overlying the calcaneum should be seen

☑ Possible # of calcaneum – consider Bohler's (see calcaneum)

kV	mAs	focus	film/screen	bucky	dose

Lateral

- Patient lies on the affected side
- Hips and knees are flexed
- Knee is supported so that the plantar aspect of the foot is at right angles to the cassette

Collimation

To include: PROXIMALLY: Calcaneum
DISTALLY: Great toe
LATERALLY: Soft tissue borders

ANKLE JOINT

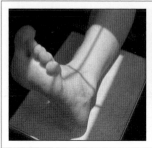
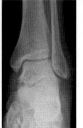

Projection: AP
Centring Point: Midway between the malleoli

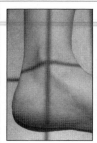
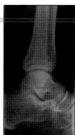

Projection: LATERAL
Centring Point: Medial malleolus

Points to consider

Technique

- ☑ AP – ankle *must* be supported in dorsiflexion
- ☑ Include calcaneum and base of fifth metatarsal
- ☑ Slight medial rotation so the head of fibula will not overlap the talus
- ☒ Stress projections – only taken under medical supervision
- ☒ Lateral – over-rotation – fibula projected too far posteriorly

kV	mAs	focus	film/screen	bucky	dose

Radiological assessment

☑ AP – widening of one side of joint space – positive injury

☑ Check fifth metatarsal – common site for #s

☑ Talus has a poor blood supply – fractured waist can result in necrosis

☑ Lateral – check calcaneum for # – the result of twisting injury

☑ Lateral – the malleoli should be superimposed

AP

- Patient seated with the ankle in dorsiflexion
- Limb rotated medially until the medial and lateral malleoli are equidistant from the cassette
- Ankle is supported by pads and sandbags

Collimation

To include: PROXIMALLY: Lower third of tibia
DISTALLY: Proximal metatarsals
LATERALLY: Soft tissue borders
MEDIALLY: Soft tissue borders

Lateral

- Patient is turned onto the side under examination
- Ankle remains in dorsiflexion and the limb is rotated until the medial and lateral malleoli are superimposed vertically
- A small pad under the toes and slight flexion of knee will aid positioning

Collimation

To include: PROXIMALLY: Lower third of tibia
DISTALLY: Calcaneum and fifth metatarsal
LATERALLY: Soft tissue borders
MEDIALLY: Soft tissue borders

CALCANEUM

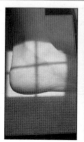 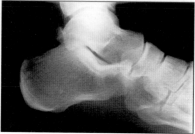

Projection: LATERAL

Centring Point: Midway between the medial malleolus and plantar aspect of the heel

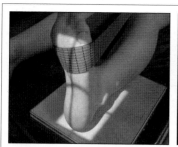 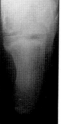

Projection: AXIAL

Centring Point: To the plantar aspect of the heel at a level 1 cm below the base of the fifth metatarsal bone. Central ray 40° caudal

Points to consider

Technique

☑ Axial – if both to be examined place a pad between heels

☑ Suspected calcaneal spur – lateral view only

☑ Vertebral # *must* be considered if a fall onto the feet

☑ Place a pad under the knee to prevent over-rotation

☑ Axial – prepare equipment first – uncomfortable for patient

kV	mAs	focus	film/screen	bucky	dose

Radiological assessment

- ☑ Suspected calcaneal # – *must* obtain an axial projection
- ☒ # of the anterior process is common – but poor visualisation of area
- ☑ Fall onto feet – associated # of upper lumbar spine (in severe cases cervical base of skull)
- ☑ Bohler's angle – if # the angle is reduced to <30°
- ☑ Sclerotic line may represent an impacted #

Lateral

- Patient lies on the side under examination
- Limb is adjusted so that the malleoli are superimposed
- A pad is placed under the knee to maintain position

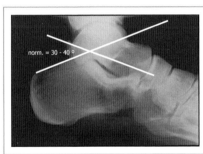

norm. = 30 - 40 °

Bohler's angle – assessed on lateral radiograph – measured by drawing a line from the posterior aspect of the calcaneum to its highest midpoint. The second line is drawn from this point to the highest anterior point. The angle is normally 30–40°

Collimation

To include: PROXIMALLY: Distal tibia/fibula
DISTALLY: Inferior calcaneum
MEDIALLY: Subtalar joints
LATERALLY: Soft tissue borders

Axial

- Patient seated with the limbs extended and the feet vertical
- Affected ankle is dorsiflexed with the aid of a bandage around the forefoot and held by the patient
- Foot is slightly internally rotated so that a line drawn down from the little toe falls to the centre of the calcaneum

Collimation

To include: SUPERIORLY: Subtalar joints
INFERIORLY: Calcaneal heel
LATERALLY: Soft tissue borders

TIBIA AND FIBULA

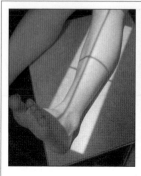 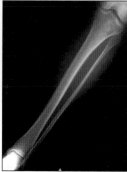

Projection: AP
Centring Point:
Midway between
the ankle and knee
joint

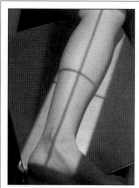 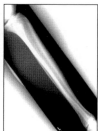

Projection: LATERAL
Centring Point: Midway
between the ankle and
knee joints

Points to consider

Technique

☑ Plantar surface of foot should be perpendicular to cassette
☑ *Must* include the knee and the ankle joint

kV	mAs	focus	film/screen	bucky	dose

☑ *Remember* – a wet plaster cast needs more exposure

☑ Tibia and fibula should be separate apart from articular ends

☒ Avoid superimposition of calcaneum and distal malleolus

☑ Lateral – horizontal beam *must* be used for acute trauma

Radiological assessment

☑ If # of the distal tibia – check proximal fibula for contrecoup #

☑ Look for subtle lucent # lines or discontinuity in trabeculae

☑ Toddler's # – child falls on one leg resulting in a spiral # of tibia – care is needed as the # may mimic vascular markings

☑ Tibia and fibula #s can compress vessels

AP

● Patient supine with the affected limb extended

● Ankle is dorsiflexed and the limb is rotated until the medial and lateral malleoli are equidistant from the cassette

● Ankle is supported by pads and sandbags

Collimation

To include: PROXIMALLY: Knee joint
DISTALLY: Ankle joint
LATERALLY: Soft tissue borders
MEDIALLY: Soft tissue borders

Lateral

● Patient is turned onto the side under examination

● Hip and knee joint are slightly flexed

● Opposite limb is moved away and supported

● Ankle remains dorsiflexed and the medial and lateral malleoli are superimposed vertically

Collimation

To include: PROXIMALLY: Knee joint
DISTALLY: Ankle joint
LATERALLY: Soft tissue borders
MEDIALLY: Soft tissue borders

KNEE JOINT

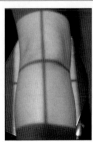 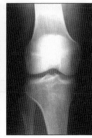

Projection: AP

Centring Point: 2.5 cm below the apex of the patella

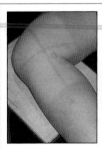 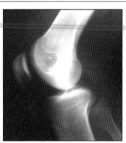

Projection: LATERAL

Centring Point: Over the superior border of the medial tibial condyle

Points to consider

Technique

☑ AP – medially rotate the lower leg 2–3°

☑ AP – to open the joint space try cephalad angle of 5°

☑ Lateral – the knee is flexed 30–40°

☑ Place a small pad under the ankle – stabilises the knee

☑ Lateral – for acute trauma you *must* use a horizontal beam

kV	mAs	focus	film/screen	bucky	dose

Radiological assessment

☑ AP – the joint spaces should be open and equidistant

☑ AP – fibula head is partially superimposed by lateral condyle

☑ Lateral – patella should be seen in profile

☑ On the horizontal beam lateral look for an articular fat-fluid level – intra-articular #

AP

- Patient supine with the affected limb extended
- Rotate the limb slightly medially to centralise the patella between the femoral condyles
- Immobilise the limb with pads and sandbags

Collimation

To include: PROXIMALLY: Patella and distal femur
DISTALLY: Proximal tibia and fibula
LATERALLY: Soft tissue borders

Lateral

- Patient is turned onto the side under examination
- Hip and knee are slightly flexed
- Unaffected limb can lie behind the affected limb or be brought well forward and supported on pads and sandbags
- Limb is rotated until the patella is at 90° to the cassette
- Raise the foot on a pad to bring the tibia parallel to the table top

Collimation

To include: PROXIMALLY: Patella and distal femur
DISTALLY: Proximal tibia and fibula
LATERALLY: Soft tissue borders

KNEE JOINT

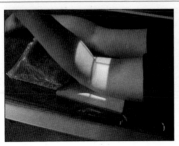 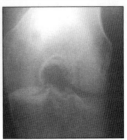

Projection: INTERCONDYLAR NOTCH – 90° ANTERIOR JOINT
Centring Point: To the crease of the knee. Central ray 90° to axis of tibia

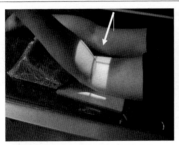 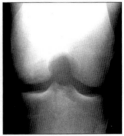

Projection: INTERCONDYLAR NOTCH – 110° POSTERIOR JOINT
Centring Point: To the crease of the knee. Central ray 110° to axis of tibia

Points to consider

Technique

☑ Anterior – ensure collimator face is parallel to the tibia
☑ Beam is angled away from the gonads
☑ Ensure the SID remains at 100 cm
☑ A single anterior projection may be sufficient
☑ If the patella apex is seen in the fossa – flex the knee more

kV	mAs	focus	film/screen	bucky	dose

Radiological assessment

☑ Useful for assessing #s of tibial spines and loose bodies

☑ Intra-articular bone fragments may indicate severe trauma and may be associated with cruciate ligament injury

☑ Two projections will be necessary to examine the whole joint

☒ Apex of the patella should not be seen within the fossa

90° anterior joint

● Patient prone on the X-ray table

● Patella should be in the centre of the femur

● Leg under examination is flexed to form an angle of approximately 60°

● Limb is supported by pads and sandbags

● Central ray perpendicular to the axis of the tibia

Collimation

Precise collimation to include the intercondylar fossa

110° posterior joint

● Patient prone on the X-ray table

● Patella should be in the centre of the femur

● Leg under examination is flexed to form an angle of approximately 60°

● Limb is supported by pads and sandbags

● Central ray should be initially 90° to the long axis of the tibia increase this angulation to 110° (i.e. angle 20° towards the femur.)

Collimation

Precise collimation to include the intercondylar fossa

KNEE JOINT

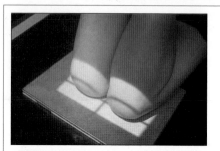

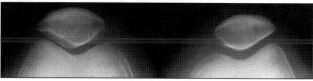

Projection: PATELLA – INFEROSUPERIOR (SKYLINE PROJECTION)

Centring Point: To the apex of the patella. Central ray adjusted to be parallel to the patella

Points to consider

Technique

- ☑ Patient prone is preferred technique
- ☑ *If* supine, place patient at the end of table – allows tube angulation
- ☒ Too much knee flexion – reduce femoropatellar joint space
- ☑ Gonad protection is *essential*
- ☒ Trauma – *do not* flex the knee – the patella may be fractured

Radiological assessment

- ☑ May demonstrate vertical #s – not seen on basic projections
- ☑ Severe muscle spasm can cause a transverse #

kV	mAs	focus	film/screen	bucky	dose

☑ Bipartite patella is normal – not to be confused with a #

☑ Look for the margins, which will be well-defined and sclerotic

Patella – inferosuperior (skyline projection)

- Patient prone
- Flex knee until patella perpendicular to table top
- Adjust leg so that there is no medial or lateral rotation
- Immobilise the lower leg with a bandage/strap placed round the ankle and held by the patient

Alternative position for skyline projection

This projection should only be used when the patient cannot lie prone and care must be taken keep the size of the field to a minimum. Gonad protection must be used.

- Patient is seated with the leg under examination flexed to form an angle of approximately 120°
- Knee supported upon pads and sandbags
- Knee is slightly medially rotated to centralise the patella between the femoral condyles
- A cassette is placed on the anterior aspect of the thigh and is angled down 15° from the vertical
- Cassette is supported in position with non-opaque pads
- Centring point: to apex of patella. Central ray angled 15° up from the horizontal, parallel with patella

Collimation

Precise collimation to include the patella and femoropatellar joint space

FEMUR

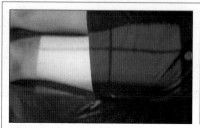 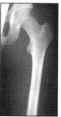

Projection: AP
Centring Point: Midway between the hip and the knee joint

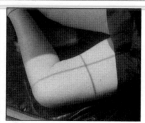 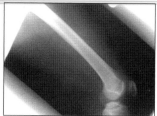

Projection: LATERAL
Centring Point: Midway between the hip and the knee joint

Points to consider

Technique

- ☑ AP – extreme care when rotating the limb
- ☑ Where possible include whole femur on one radiograph
- ☑ Use gonad shielding – take care not to occlude area of interest
- ☒ Divergent beam – take care not to project hip or knee off cassette
- ☒ Lateral is *not* recommended if there may be a #
- ☑ Use horizontal beam to obtain lateral if query #

kV	mAs	focus	film/screen	bucky	dose

Radiological assessment

☑ #ed shaft of femur – the result of considerable force

☑ Look for limb shortening and displacement

☑ Fracture causes considerable loss of blood – consider patient in shock

☑ # completely intra-articular – the bones may not unite

☑ Symptoms of a fractured pubic ramus can mimic those of a #ed femoral neck

☑ If hip and knee joint not included on one image – take hip down on one projection and knee up on the other – as demonstrated on the radiographs

AP

● Patient supine with the leg under examination extended

● Where possible gently rotate the limb medially to centralise the patella between the femoral condyles

● Immobilise with pads and sandbags to maintain position

Collimation

To include: PROXIMALLY: Hip joint
DISTALLY: Knee joint
LATERALLY: Soft tissue borders
MEDIALLY: Soft tissue borders

Lateral

● Patient turns onto the side under examination with the hip and knee slightly flexed

● Pelvis is slightly rotated away from the leg under examination to separate the two thighs and visualise the upper femur

● Affected limb is adjusted so that the femoral condyles are superimposed

● Immobilise with pads and sandbags to maintain position

Collimation

To include: PROXIMALLY: Hip joint
DISTALLY: Knee joint
LATERALLY: Soft tissue borders
MEDIALLY: Soft tissue borders

FEMUR

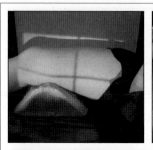 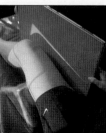

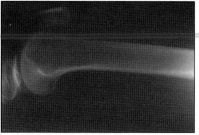

Projection: LATERAL – HORIZONTAL BEAM

Centring Point: Midway between the hip and knee joint. Horizontal central ray

Points to consider

Technique

☑ Use if there may be a fractured femur or patient cannot turn onto their side

☑ For upper femur – cassette on lateral side of the thigh

☑ For lower femur – cassette against medial side of the thigh

☑ Use gonad shielding – take care not to occlude area of interest

☒ *Do not* rotate the limb – this will exacerbate the injury

kV	mAs	focus	film/screen	bucky	dose

Radiological assessment

☑ Check for any break in the cortical outline

☑ Remember symptoms of a fractured pubic ramus can mimic those of a fractured neck of femur

☑ Femoral condylar #s can be displaced or undisplaced

☑ Severe comminuted condylar #s may be associated with a spiral # of the distal femur

Lateral – horizontal beam

Medio-lateral

● Patient supine

● Leg under examination is extended

● Rotate the limb to centralise the patella over the femur

● Opposite limb is raised upon a suitable support and is immobilised

● Cassethe supported vertically on lateral aspect of thigh under examination

Collimation

To include: PROXIMALLY: Upper femur
             DISTALLY: Knee joint
             LATERALLY: Soft tissue borders
             MEDIALLY: Soft tissue borders

NB

Latero-medial projection

Support cassette on the medical aspect of the affected limb. Useful when the patient is unable to raise the leg not being examined.

8 Vertebral Column

CERVICAL SPINE

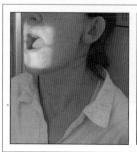 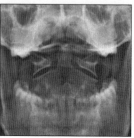

Projection: AP
C1–C3

Centring Point:
To the lower border
of the incisors –
directly to the open
mouth

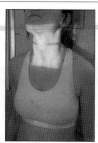 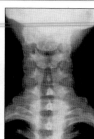

Projection: AP C3–C7

Centring Point: To the sternal
notch – then angle the central ray
cranially to the thyroid cartilage.
Central ray approximately 15°
cranially

Points to consider

Technique

- ☑ Remember to set the exposure before positioning
- ☑ Remember to remove jewelry that is in the field of interest and dentures/
  orthodontic appliances where possible
- ☑ AP C1–C3 – adjust patient so that occipital bone and lower edge of upper
  incisors are superimposed
- ☒ AP C1–C3 – patient may overextend the head when opening the mouth
- ☑ AP – mental region of mandible should be superimposed over the occiput

kV	mAs	focus	film/screen	bucky	dose

Radiological assessment

☑ Check that each intervertebral joint space is consistent

☑ AP C1–C3 – the odontoid process *must* be clear of the occipital bone

☑ All vertebral bodies should be rectangular – any variation may be due to trauma

☑ AP – ensure C3–T1 are visualised – C1–C3 may be obscured

AP C1–C3

● Patient erect or supine

● Median sagittal plane 90° to the cassette

● Patient's neck is extended until the upper occlusal plane is perpendicular to the table top

● The patient is then asked to open the mouth as wide as possible, ensure the occlusal plane remains perpendicular to the table top

Collimation

To include: SUPERIORLY: Upper C1
INFERIORLY: Body C3
LATERALLY: Transverse processes

AP C3–C7

● Patient erect or supine

● Median sagittal plane 90° to the cassette

● Patient's neck is extended until the angle of the mouth and the tragus of the ear are perpendicular to the table top

Collimation

To include: SUPERIORLY: Lower border of mandible
INFERIORLY: Body T1
LATERALLY: Transverse processes

CERVICAL SPINE

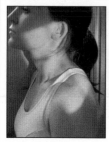 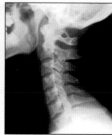

Projection: LATERAL
Centring Point: 2.5 cm behind and 5 cm below the angle of the mandible

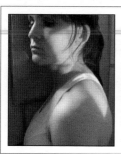 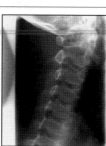

Projection: ANTERIOR OBLIQUES
Centring Point: To the middle of the cervical spine. Central ray 15° caudal

Points to consider

Technique

☑ Acute trauma – use horizontal beam – *do not* adjust head

☑ Remember to remove jewelry/ear-rings that is in the field of interest

☑ Exposure made on arrested expiration

☑ *Must* include C7 on the radiograph

☑ Oblique – extend the head back to avoid superimposition of the mandible

kV	mAs	focus	film/screen	bucky	dose

Radiological assessment

☑ Anterior displacement over 3.5 mm – ligaments torn

☑ Vertebral bodies C3–T1 should be the same size – a disparity of 2 mm may be due to a compression #

☑ Check all seven vertebrae are seen on the radiograph

☑ Oblique – demonstrates intervertebral foramina closest to the film (right anterior oblique – right foramina; left anterior oblique – left foramina)

Lateral

● Patient in the erect position with the shoulder against the cassette

● Median sagittal plane parallel to the cassette

● Patient's shoulders should be relaxed and arms are placed down and slightly behind the trunk

● Feet are separated to aid stability

● Patient's chin is raised and extended slightly forwards so that the mandible does not obscure the spine

Collimation

To include: SUPERIORLY: EAM
INFERIORLY: Body T1
LATERALLY: Soft tissue borders

Anterior obliques – both sides for comparison

● Patient erect facing a vertical bucky

● Trunk is then rotated 45° to each side in turn

● Patient's head is rotated so that the median sagittal plane is parallel to the bucky

● As with every x-ray ensure anatomical legends are applied as interpretation without them at times can be confusing

Collimation

To include: SUPERIORLY: EAM
INFERIORLY: Body T1
LATERALLY: Soft tissue borders

CERVICOTHORACIC

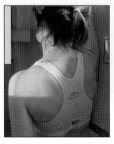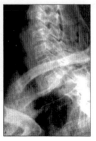

Projection: SWIMMER'S

Centring Point: To a level just above the shoulder remote from the cassette. Horizontal central ray

Points to consider

Technique

- ☑ Remember to set the exposure before positioning
- ☑ Exposure *must* penetrate the shoulder region
- ☒ *Do not* rotate the thorax unless an oblique projection is required
- ☑ Exposure on *arrested* respiration

Radiological assessment

- ☑ Check that each intervertebral joint space is consistent
- ☑ Shoulders should be seen separated from each other
- ☑ All vertebral bodies should be rectangular – any variation may be due to trauma
- ☑ *Must* include from C5 to T5

Swimmer's

- Patient erect
- Shoulder is placed against the erect bucky

kV	mAs	focus	film/screen	bucky	dose

- Arm nearest the cassette is raised and folded over the head
- Arm furthest from the cassette is depressed as far as possible
- Median sagittal plane is parallel to the cassette

Collimation

To include: SUPERIORLY: Body C5
INFERIORLY: Body T5
ANTERIORLY: Anterior clavicles
POSTERIORLY: Posterior ribs

THORACIC SPINE

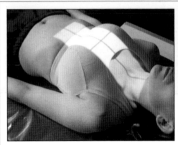 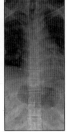

Projection: AP
Centring Point: To a point 5 cm below the suprasternal notch

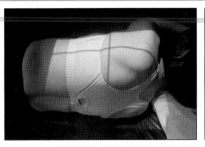 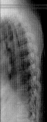

Projection: LATERAL
Centring Point: To a point 5 cm anterior to the palpable sixth spinous process

Points to consider

Technique

☑ AP – use a wedge filter to prevent the upper thoracic vertebrae being over-penetrated

☑ Flex the knees to aid the patient's comfort

☑ AP – exposure on arrested inspiration

☑ Lateral – a long exposure with gentle breathing to blur the lung fields and ribs (diffusion technique)

kV	mAs	focus	film/screen	bucky	dose

Radiological assessment

☑ AP – abnormal soft tissue enlargement around the spine is a positive indication of trauma or infection

☑ Check all pedicles are present and intact

☑ Vertebral bodies should be the same height – anteriorly and posteriorly

☑ Lateral – upper spine difficult to visualise due to shoulders. A swimmer's projection may be required – CT is better

AP

- Patient supine
- Median sagittal plane perpendicular to the cassette
- A small pillow supports the head
- Patient's arms are placed down by the side

Collimation

To include: SUPERIORLY: Body of C7
                INFERIORLY: Body of L1
                LATERALLY: Transverse processes and soft tissues

Lateral

- Patient lying on their side
- Median sagittal plane and the spine are parallel to the table top
- Arms are raised and placed onto the pillow
- Knees are flexed and a soft pad is placed between them for comfort

Collimation

To include: SUPERIORLY: Upper thoracic spine
                INFERIORLY: Body of L1
                ANTERIORLY: Vertebral bodies
                POSTERIORLY: Posterior rib cage

LUMBAR SPINE

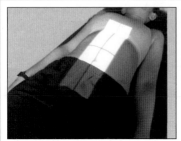
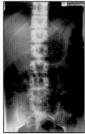

Projection: AP

Centring Point: Midline at the level of lower costal margin

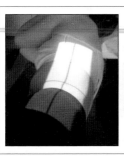
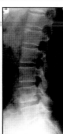

Projection: LATERAL

Centring Point: 8–10 cm anterior to the third lumbar spinous process at the level of the lower costal margin

Points to consider

Technique

☑ AP – reduce lumbar lordosis – flex knees and support where indicated

☑ AP – ensure sacroiliac joints included on the radiograph

☑ AP and lateral – exposure on arrested *expiration* – diaphragm should be above L1 – or try breathing technique to blur bowel shadows

☑ Lateral – non-opaque pad under the waist may assist in bringing the spine parallel to the table top

☑ Use gonad shield – but take care not to obscure the area of interest

kV	mAs	focus	film/screen	bucky	dose

Radiological assessment

☑ AP – distance between pedicles gradually widens from L1 to L5

☑ AP – *must* inspect the transverse processes for #

☑ Check soft tissue changes – may indicate underlying pathology – renal stones mimic skeletal back pain

☑ Lateral – vertebral bodies should be same height anteriorly and posteriorly

☑ Any loss of height or wedging suggests a possible compression #

AP

- Patient supine
- Median sagittal plane perpendicular to the table top and the anterior superior iliac spines (ASIS) are equidistant
- Hips and knees are flexed and where indicated supported with pads
- Patient's arms are placed across the upper thorax or away from the body

Collimation

To include: SUPERIORLY: T12
INFERIORLY: Sacroiliac joints
(Some imaging centres require visualisation of the kidneys due to the possibility of referred pain from kidney pathology)
LATERALLY: Sacroiliac joints

Lateral

- Patient lying on side
- Median sagittal plane and the spine are parallel to the table top
- Arms are raised and placed onto the pillow
- Knees are flexed and a soft pad may be placed between them for comfort

Collimation

To include: SUPERIORLY: T12
INFERIORLY: L5 – sacral junction
ANTERIORLY: Vertebral bodies (possibly kidneys)
POSTERIORLY: Spinous processes

LUMBAR SPINE

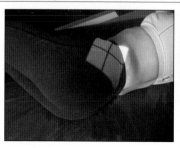 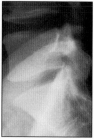

Projection: LUMBOSACRAL JUNCTION (L5–S1)

Centring Point: 8 cm anterior to the fifth lumbar spinous process

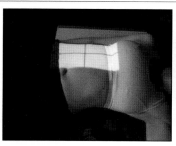 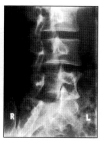

Projection: AP OBLIQUES

Centring Point: To the mid-clavicular line on the raised side at the level of lower costal margin

Points to consider

Technique

☑ *Do not* proceed until you have examined the lateral

☑ L5–S1 – a 5° caudal angulation may open the disc space

kV	mAs	focus	film/screen	bucky	dose

☑ L5–S1 – collimation important to reduce scattered radiation

☑ Lateral – place a non-opaque pad under the waist to bring the spine parallel to the table top

Radiological assessment

☑ Disc space at L5–S1 – usually smaller than at L4–L5

☑ Joint space *must* be visualised open

☑ Obliques – suspected spondylolisthesis – a defect in pars articularis – look for a collar around the Scottie dog's neck!

☑ Obliques – will demonstrate superior and inferior articular processes and the zygopophyseal joints of the side nearest the cassette

Lumbosacral junction (L5–S1)

● Patient lying on side

● Median sagittal plane and the spine are parallel to the table top

● Arms are raised and placed onto the pillow

● Knees are flexed and a soft pad may be placed between them for comfort

● Posterior superior iliac spines (PSIS) are perpendicular to the table top

Collimation

To include: SUPERIORLY: L5
              INFERIORLY: Sacral segment
              ANTERIORLY: Anterior lumbar bodies
              POSTERIORLY: Spinous processes

AP obliques

● Patient supine

● Trunk is rotated 45° to either side in turn

● Hips and knees are flexed and supported in position

Collimation

To include: SUPERIORLY: L1
              INFERIORLY: Upper sacral segment
              LATERALLY: Spinal column

SACRUM

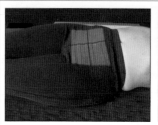 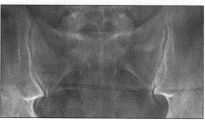

Projection: AP

Centring Point: Midline 5 cm above superior border of symphysis pubis. Cranial – central ray: 10° male, 20° female

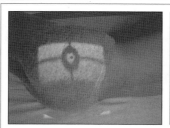 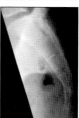

Projection: LATERAL

Centring Point: Midway between the PSIS and the palpable coccyx

Points to consider

Technique

☑ AP – lower bowel preparation is an advantage

☑ AP – central ray will differ between males and females

☑ Lateral – where indicated place a non-opaque pad under the waist

kV	mAs	focus	film/screen	bucky	dose

Radiological assessment

☑ *Must* demonstrate the sacrum and sacroiliac joints

☑ Obturator foramina will appear wide open

☑ Symphysis will appear broadened depending upon tube angle

☑ Lateral – *must* include the L5–S1 joint space on the radiograph

AP

● Patient supine

● Median sagittal plane perpendicular to the table top and ASIS equidistant

● Hips and knees are flexed and may be supported in position

Collimation

To include: SUPERIORLY: L5–S1 joint space
              INFERIORLY: Coccyx
              LATERALLY: Sacroiliac joints

Lateral

● Patient lies on their side

● Median sagittal plane parallel to the table top

● Hips and knees are flexed

● PSIS are perpendicular to the table top

Collimation

To include: SUPERIORLY: L5–S1 joint space
              INFERIORLY: Coccyx
              ANTERIORLY: Sacral promontory and coccyx
              POSTERIORLY: Sacral spinous tubercles

9

The Skull

SKULL BASELINES

Orbitomeatal baseline

Line joins the outer canthus of the eye to the midpoint of the external auditory meatus

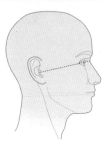

Anthropological baseline

Line joins the infraorbital margin to the superior border of the external auditory meatus.
The difference in angles between the *orbitomeatal baseline* and the *anthropological baseline* is 10°

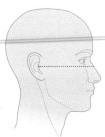

Auricular line

Line passes perpendicular to the anthropological baseline through the centre of the external auditory meatus

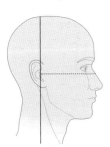

Interpupillary line

Line joins the centre of the two orbits and is perpendicular to the median sagittal plane

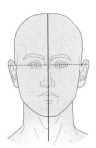

Notes:

ISOCENTRIC TECHNIQUE

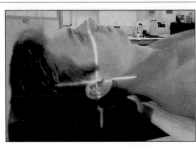

Reference position

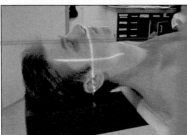

Facial bones reference position

☑ *Total* immobilisation of the patient is essential

☑ Patient can be examined erect or supine – easier to immobilise when supine

☑ Overexposure can be tolerated more than underexposure

☑ Dulac technique is positioning patient so that the area of interest is in the centre of a sphere – *isocentre*

☒ Unsure of your position – move the tube 180° to check the other side

☑ Up to 50% reduction in dose can be achieved

☑ Radiation protection – use cones and collimators to limit the beam – *most important* – to avoid the need for repeats

☑ Some radiographs may appear different – due to decrease in distortion and true representation of the patient

kV	mAs	focus	film/screen	bucky	dose

☑ Skull #s – linear is most common – stellate is star shaped.

☑ Depressed – detached fragment and may be comminuted

☑ Where possible the patient should remain in a comfortable position – different projections achieved by moving the tube

Planes

● Median sagittal plane = Vertical

● Anthropological plane = Vertical

● Auricular plane = Horizontal

Reference position

● Patient supine

● Head resting on non-opaque pad over the head support

Tube column

● Tube and vertical arm is set to 0° so that it is perpendicular to the table top

● Sagittal light beam should coincide with median sagittal plane and the transverse light beam with the anthropological plane

● Horizontal beam *must* pass through auditory canals and coincide with auricular plane

● Velcro band placed across the forehead to maintain this position

Main movements

● Above (vent: ventral) and below (dors: dorsal)

  – Degree of displacement in relation to the auricular plane, e.g. vent 4 cm = tube *raised* 4 cm *above* the *auricular* plane

  – Dors 4 cm = tube *lowered* 4 cm *below* the *auricular* plane

● Right and left

  – Degree of displacement in relation to the median sagittal plane, e.g. moving the patient to the left brings the right half of the skull into the isocentre

● Cranial and caudal

  – Patient displacement in relation to the anthropological plane

ISOCENTRIC TECHNIQUE

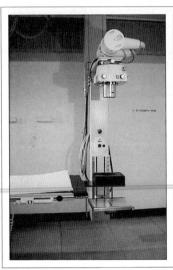
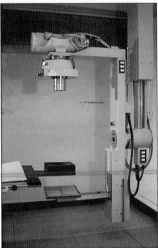

Reminder

Lateral position

Tube positioned lateral to the patient so that the tube can be rotated cephalad or caudad along the long axis of the table and patient

Medial position

Tube positioned so that the column is at the vertex of the skull so that the tube can be angled to either side of the head

Basic equipment positions

- Lateral – L
  - Tube arm and vertical arm at 0°
  - 'C' arm at the side of the patient's head
  - Used to set the reference position and examination area

kV	mAs	focus	film/screen	bucky	dose

- Medial – M
  - 'C' arm supporting the tube is parallel to the median sagittal plane
  - X-ray tube is able to be rotated laterally to either side of the patient's head
  - Used to rotate the tube and for lateral projections

Magnification

Should be kept the same for all projections (1, 2)

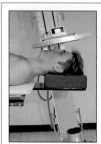 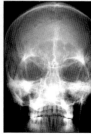

Projection: OCCIPITOFRONTAL
Central ray: Directed 10° caudad.
Entry point: Midline between parietal
bones. Exit point: Nasion

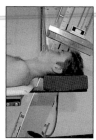 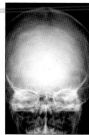

Projection: PINEAL
Central ray: Directed 25° cephalad.
Entry point: 2 cm above external
occipital protuberance. Exit point:
4 cm above the glabella

Occipitofrontal

☑ Visualise – anterior vault – frontal sinuses – facial bones
☑ Correct position:

- Measure outer orbit to the lateral vault on both sides
- Petrous ridge should be level with the lower orbital margin

☒ If petrous ridge is below lower orbital margin the angle is too great – if it
appears within the orbits the angle is too small

kV	mAs	focus	film/screen	bucky	dose

Pineal

☑ Visualise – the pineal gland's position within the vault

☑ Correct position:

- Distance from the outer orbital margin should be symmetrical on both sides
- Petrous ridges and orbital margins should be superimposed and anterior clinoid processes should be at the same level

☒ If petrous ridge is below orbital margin the angle is too small – if it appears above the orbits the angle is too great

Occipitofrontal

- Tube column base position: lateral, with X-ray tube beneath the patient
- Patient displacement: caudad 4 cm (brings nasion and frontal structures to the isocentre)

Pineal

- Tube column base position: lateral, with X-ray tube beneath the patient
- Patient displacement: caudad 4 cm (to bring the pineal gland to the isocentre)

SKULL

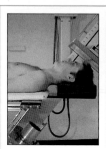 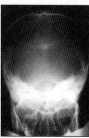

Projection: HALF-AXIAL

Central ray: Directed 40° cephalad. Entry point: Midline through foramen magnum. Exit point: Midline 6 cm above glabella

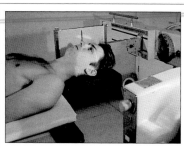 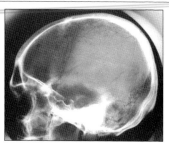

Projection: LATERAL

Central ray: Horizontal. Entry point: 4 cm above the anthropological baseline in the auricular plane. Exit point: Corresponds to opposite side

Half-axial

☑ Visualise – occiput – foramen magnum – lambdoid suture

☑ Correct position:

- Not easy to assess – middle of foramen magnum should be equidistant to the outer skull on both sides – posterior clinoid processes seen within the foramen magnum

☒ Too little angle – foramen magnum will not be seen

kV	mAs	focus	film/screen	bucky	dose

Lateral

☑ Visualise – whole of the vault – some facial bones – mandible

☑ Correct position:

- Superimposed is the anterior cranial fossa – middle fossa – external auditory meatus (EAM)
- Posterior rami of the mandible

☒ If EAM is separated the head is rotated – if the anterior cranial fossa is separated the head is tilted

Half-axial

- Tube column base position: lateral, with X-ray tube beneath the patient
- Patient displacement: caudad 4 cm

Lateral

Horizontal beam is imperative

- Tube column base position: medial, tube at the side of the patient's head so the central ray is horizontal
- Patient displacement: caudad 4 cm

FACIAL BONES

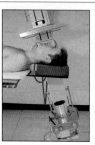 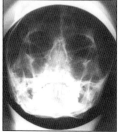

Projection: OCCIPITOMENTAL 15°

Central ray: Directed 15° caudad. Entry point: The occipital bone. Exit point: Upper incisor teeth

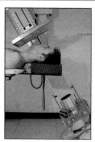 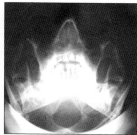

Projection: OCCIPITOMENTAL 30°

Central ray: Directed 30° caudad. Entry point: The occipital bone. Exit point: Upper incisor teeth

Occipitomental 15°

☑ Visualise – maxilla – zygoma – lower orbital margin

☑ Correct position:

- Petrous bone just below the apex of the maxillary sinuses
- Distance from outer orbital margin should be symmetrical on both sides

☑ Erect technique for blow-out # of the floor of the orbit

kV	mAs	focus	film/screen	bucky	dose

Occipitomental 30°

☑ Visualise – orbital floor – zygomatic arch
☑ Correct position:
  ● Petrous bone level with the body of the mandible
  ● Distance from outer orbital margin should be symmetrical on both sides
☑ Erect technique for blow-out # of the floor of the orbit

Occipitomental 15°

● Tube column base position: lateral, with X-ray tube beneath the patient
● Tube displacement: 6 cm above the auricular plane
● Patient position: patient's anthropological baseline is raised 30°

Occipitomental 30°

● Tube column base position: lateral, with X-ray tube beneath the patient
● Tube displacement: 6 cm above the auricular plane
● Patient position: patient's anthropological baseline is raised 30°

NON-ISOCENTRIC TECHNIQUE

Skull radiography not using isocentric equipment

Where possible the projections should be taken PA to reduce radiation dose to the eyes

Projection	Patient position	Orbitomeatal baseline/ OM line to table top	Median sagittal plane to table top	Centring point/tube angulation	Additional comments
Occipitofrontal	Prone	90°	90°	In the midline through the occipital bone to the glabella with a straight tube	Petrous ridges demonstrated within the orbits
Occipitofrontal 20°	Prone	90°	90°	In the midline through the occipital bone to the nasion with 20° cranio-caudal angulation	Demonstrates the frontal bone and the roof of the orbits. The petrous ridge projects just into the lower orbital rim
Fronto-occipital	Supine	90°	90°	In the midline to the glabella with a straight tube	Petrous ridges demonstrated within the orbits
Fronto-occipital 30°/ half-axial/ Townes	Supine	90°	90°	2.5 cm above the glabella 30° cranio-caudal angulation	Demonstrates the occipital bone, the dorsum sellae within the foramen magnum. Petrous and mastoid portions of the temporal bone
Lateral	Prone, oblique, head turned to side		Parallel	2.5 cm cranial to the EAM (external auditory meatus)	Infraorbital line 90° to the table top. Adjust centring point anterior-posterior to ensure that both the frontal and occipital bone are included
Lateral with horizontal beam	Supine		Parallel	2.5 cm cranial to the EAM with horizontal beam	Infraorbital line 90° to the cassette. Small radiolucent pad under the head to ensure that the occipital bone is included. Demonstrates fluid levels – sphenoid sinus, air in the cranial cavity
Facial bones mento- occipital 20°	Supine	Raised 45°	90°	In the midline to base of the nasal septum just above the upper lip with a 20° caudo-cranial angulation	Demonstrates facial bones and maxillary sinuses clear of the petrous ridge. Where the patient cannot raise the chin to give an OM line of 45° the tube angle must be increased

Appendix

FURTHER PROJECTIONS

Location	Projection	Exposure	Notes

Location	Projection	Exposure	Notes

EXPOSURE FACTORS

In selecting the exposure factors for an examination the radiographer is attempting to produce an image of optimum quality but at minimum radiation dose to the patient. Below is a summary of some of the factors which might be changed and their direct and indirect effect(s) on image quality and radiation dose to the patient.

Factor increased ↑	Effect on the radiation beam leaving the tube	Direct effect on image quality	Indirect effect on image quality	Effect on radiation dose to the patient
mAs ↑	Quantity ↑	Image darker	May require larger focal spot to allow increased time	Dose ↑
kVp ↑	Quality ↑ Quantity ↑	Contrast ↓ Density ↑	Lower mAs	Less dose to area – gonad ↑
Collimation (tightened)	Smaller area no effect on quality/ quantity	Improves contrast	Needs mAs ↑	Reduces dose ↓
SID	No effect	Alters magnification OID/SOD ratio	Requires mAs ↑	Slight reduction ↓
Use of secondary radiation grid	No effect	Contrast ↑	Requires mAs ↑	Dose ↑
Altering the speed class sharpness of the film/screen combination	No effect	Increase photographic	Requires mAs ↓	Reduced ↓

GLOSSARY OF COMMON MEDICAL TERMS

Abortion – Natural or artificial expulsion from uterus
Abscess – Localised collection of pus
Achalasia – Obstruction due to non-relaxant muscular sphincter
Achondroplasia – Dwarfism due to the failure of endochondral ossification
Acoustic neuroma – Benign tumour of the eighth cranial nerve
Acromegaly – Overgrowth of soft and bony structures, result of pituitary tumour
Addison's disease – Chronic adrenal cortical failure associated with adults
Adenoma – Benign tumour of glandular tissues
Adhesions – Fibrous tissue bands due to inflammation or surgery
Akathisia – The inability to sit still associated with Parkinson's disease
Albuminuria – Albumin found in the urine
Alopecia – Baldness
Alport's syndrome – Albuminuria associated with deafness and eye lesions
Aluminosis – Lung fibrosis due to inhalation of metallic dust
Amenorrhoea – Absence of menstrual periods
Anencephaly – Congenital absence of cranial vault and brain
Aneurysm – Localised distension of an artery or duct
Angioma – Benign tumour associated with blood vessels
Ankylosing spondylitis – Arthritis of the spine resulting in fusion of the vertebrae
Ankylosis – Immobilisation of a joint
Antepartum – Before delivery
Aortic regurgitation – Blood backflow through the aortic valve of the heart
Aortic stenosis – Narrowing of the aortic valve
Arachnodactyly – Abnormally long fingers or toes
Areflexia – Absence of reflexes
Arteriosclerosis – Hardening of the arteries with narrowing of the lumen
Arthrodesis – Surgical fusion of a joint
Asbestosis – Lung disease due to exposure to dust (asbestos)
Ascites – Excess fluid in the peritoneum
Asthenia – Generalised and non-specific weakness
Astrocytoma – A cranial tumour – the commonest form of glioma
Atelectasis – Collapse or non-expansion of the lungs
Atheroma – Fatty degeneration of inner linings of blood vessels
Atherosclerosis – Arterial disease with atheroma
Atresia – Failure of normal lumen to develop in hollow organs
Atrophy – Abnormal reduction in the size of tissues
Auricular fibrillation – Abnormality in the rhythm of heart beat
Avulsion – The forcible tearing away of bone fragments

Benign – Non-malignant, simple tumour
Bennett's fracture – Fracture of the base of the thumb involving the joint
Brachycephaly – A short high skull associated with premature suture closure
Bright's disease – Kidney disease, a form of nephritis
Bronchiectasis – Dilatation of the bronchi, often associated with infection
Bursa – Pocket-like structure containing a small quantity of fluid
Bursitis – Inflammation of a bursa

Calculus – A stone
Callus – Temporary bone formed during the process of healing
Carcinoma – A malignant tumour of epithelial origin
Carcinomatosis – Diffuse spread of carcinoma
Carditis – Inflammation of the heart
Cellulitis – Spreading infection of connective tissue
Cholecystectomy – Surgical removal of the gallbladder
Cholecystitis – Inflammation of the gallbladder

Cholelithiasis – Formation of stones within the gallbladder or ducts
Chondroma – A benign tumour of cartilage
Chondromalacia patellae – Juvenile osteoarthritis-like condition of the knee
Chordoma – Rare locally malignant tumour of the skull or sacral region
Claudication – Deficient blood supply, intermittent pain on exertion
Coarctation – Congenital narrowing in the thoracic aorta
Coeliac disease – Malabsorption and gluten sensitivity associated with loss of villi
Colostrum – High protein milk produced in the first days of lactation
Congenital – Present at birth
Congestion – Accumulation of fluid in the body tissues
Consolidation – Solidification of exudate, usually in the lungs
Contusion – Bruising
Coxa vara – Congenital deformity of the neck of femur
Craniostenosis – Premature closure of cranial sutures
Crepitus – The sound and feel of a fracture or surfaces rubbing together
Crohn's disease – Chronic non-specific inflammation of any part of intestine
Croup – Infant cough with dyspnoea due to mucosal swelling
Cushing's syndrome – Effect of excess adrenal corticosteroids
Cyanosis – Bluish skin caused by insufficient oxygenation
Cyst – Hollow sac containing fluid or semi-solid material

Dacryoadenitis – Inflammation of the lacrimal glands
Degloving – Traumatic detachment of the skin from underlying tissues
Dermoid cyst – Cystic structure containing fluid and semi-solid material
Dextrocardia – The siting of the heart on the right side of the thorax
Diabetes mellitus – High blood sugar due to a deficiency of insulin
Diaphysis – The shaft of a long bone
Dislocation – Displacement of the bones that form a joint
Diverticulitis – Inflammation of the diverticula of the bowel
Diverticulosis – Presence of numerous diverticula in the bowel
Diverticulum – Abnormal outpouching arising from a hollow organ
Ductus arteriosus patent – Failure of the ductus arteriosus to close after birth
Dysmenorrhoea – Painful menstrual periods
Dyspepsia – Indigestion
Dysphagia – Difficulty in swallowing
Dysphasia – Speech defect due to cerebral cortical mechanisms
Dysplasia – Abnormality of growth
Dyspnoea – Difficulty in breathing
Dystrophy – Abnormal bone growth associated with poor nutrition
Dysuria – Difficult and or painful micturition

Ectopic pregnancy – Fetus formed outside the uterus
Effusion – Formation of fluid within a body cavity
Embolism – Obstruction of blood flow by a blood clot or other matter
Emphysema – Excessive size of lung alveoli due to prolonged stress
Empyema – Abscess containing pus within an enclosed cavity
Encephalitis – Inflammation of the brain
Enchondroma – Benign tumour of cartilage growing within bone
Endocarditis – Inflammation of the endocardium of the heart
Enteritis – Regional inflammation of the intestine
Enuresis – Urinary incontinence
Epilepsy – Episodic disorder of brain function producing a fit
Epistaxis – Nose bleed
Epithelioma – Tumour derived from epithelial cells
Ewing's sarcoma – Small cell carcinoma affecting juvenile bones
Exacerbation – Increase in severity
Exostosis – Outgrowth of bone

Fibrillation – Rapid and irregular movements of muscle fibres
Fibroid – Simple tumour of the uterus
Fistula – Abnormal communication between organs
Flail chest – Multiple rib fractures producing paradoxical movement of the chest wall
Freiberg's disease – Aseptic necrosis of metatarsal head, usually the second

Galeazzi's fracture – Fracture of radius with dislocation of radial head
Gangrene – Tissue necrosis due to lack of blood supply
Glioma – General term for tumour of nervous system
Glycosuria – Sugar in the urine
Goitre – Enlargement of the thyroid
Gout – Disease due to excess uric acid in the blood
Grand mal – Epilepsy with classic epileptic fits
Gravid – Pregnant woman
Greenstick fracture – Partial fracture or bending of children's bones
Guillain–Barré syndrome – Acute disorder with loss of conduction in peripheral nerves associated with respiratory difficulty

Haemangioma – Tumour of vascular tissues
Haematemesis – Vomiting of blood
Haematuria – Blood in the urine
Haemoptysis – Coughing-up of blood
Hallux valgus – Deviation of the big toe towards the other toes
Hemiplegia – Paralysis of one side of the body
Hepatitis – Inflammation of the liver
Hernia – Abnormal protrusion of tissue through any orifice
Hiatus hernia – Protrusion of abdominal organ through the diaphragm
Hirschsprung's disease – Congenital absence of muscle layer in the colon
Hodgkin's disease – Disease of the lymphatic system
Hydatid cyst – Cyst formed by infestation of a tapeworm
Hydrocephalus – Excess cerebrospinal fluid within the skull vault
Hydronephrosis – Enlargement of the kidney due to obstruction
Hydropneumothorax – The presence of fluid and air in the pleural cavity
Hydrothorax – The presence of fluid in the pleural cavity
Hyperglycaemia – Excessive sugar in the bloodstream
Hypernephroma – Carcinoma of the renal parenchyma
Hyperplasia – Tissue enlargement, without neoplasia
Hypertension – Abnormal high blood pressure
Hypertrophy – Enlargement of an organ through increase in tissue
Hypoplasia – Underdevelopment

Idiopathic – A disease of unknown origin
Ileitis – Inflammation of the ileum
Ileostomy – Artificial opening of the ileum onto the abdominal wall
Ileus – Intestinal obstruction
Infarction – Death of cells due to termination of blood supply
Inflammation – A local reaction of the body's cells to damage or infection
Intussusception – Obstruction in infants due to invagination of part of gut into a lower segment
Ischaemia – Local inadequacy of blood supply

Jaundice – Yellowing of skin due to excessive bilirubin in the blood

Kienböck's disease – Aseptic necrosis of lunate bone
Klippel–Feil syndrome – Congenital short neck with fusion of vertebrae
Köhler's disease – Aseptic necrosis of navicular bone
Kyphosis – Excessive backward convexity of the spine

Laminectomy – Surgical approach to the cord by removal of lamina
Lesion – Any injury or damage to tissue
Leukaemia – Malignant disease of blood, excessive production of white cells
Lipoma – Benign tumour developing from fat cells
Lordosis – Excessive forward convexity of the spine
Lumbago – Local pain arising from the lumbar spine
Lymphoma – Tumour of the lymphoid tissues

Malaise – A general feeling of being unwell
Malignant – Life-threatening tumour producing secondary effects
Mastectomy – Surgical removal of the breast
Mastoidectomy – Surgical operation on the mastoid air cells
Meckel's diverticulum – Outpouching of ileal wall, rudimentary remains of a duct
Megacolon – Dilation of the colon associated with constipation
Melaena – Faeces blackened by blood
Melanoma – Tumour of melanocytes, which are pigment-producing cells in the skin
Menière's disease – Disease of the inner ear associated with tinnitus and vertigo
Meninges – Membranes covering the brain and spinal cord
Meningioma – Generally benign tumour of the meninges
Meningitis – Inflammation of the meninges
Meningocoele – Congenital herniation of meninges through the skull or cord
Meniscectomy – Surgical removal of cartilage from the knee joint
Menorrhagia – Excessive loss of blood during menstrual periods
Multigravida – Woman with one or more previous pregnancies
Multipara – Woman who has given birth to one or more children
Mumps – An acute infection of the parotid salivary gland
Myasthenia gravis – Disease associated with voluntary muscle weakness
Myeloma – Tumour of bone marrow, characterised by multiple tumours
Myocarditis – Inflammation of the myocardium
Myositis ossificans – Ossification of a haematoma over bone following trauma

Naevus – A birth mark or mole on the skin
Necrosis – Death of an organ or tissue within a living body
Neoplasm – A tumour that can be benign or malignant
Nephrectomy – The surgical removal of a kidney
Nephritis – Inflammation of the kidney
Nephrostomy – Surgical drainage of the kidney
Neuralgia – Pain arising from the nervous system
Neuroblastoma – Malignant tumour in children arising from adrenal medulla
Neurofibroma – Benign tumour arising from the fibrous sheath of a nerve

Oedema – Increase in fluid within the tissues
Oesophageal varices – Dilated veins of the lower oesophagus associated with portal hypertension
Osgood–Schlatter – Osteochondritis of the tibial tubercle disease
Osteitis – Inflammation of bone
Osteoarthritis – Chronic degenerative arthritis
Osteochondroma – Benign tumour composed of bone and cartilage
Osteoclastoma – Bone tumour associated with long bone ends in young adults
Osteogenesis imperfecta – Defect of bone formation, with fragile easily fractured bones
Osteoma – Benign bone tumour associated with the skull or facial bones
Osteomalacia – Defective calcification of bone due to vitamin D deficiency
Osteomyelitis – Inflammation of bone
Osteoporosis – Loss of bone tissue with inadequate new replacement
Otalgia – Pain in the ear
Otitis media – Inflammation of the middle ear
Otorrhoea – A discharge from the ear

Paget's disease – Chronic disease of bone associated with softening and deformity
Pancreatitis – Inflammation of the pancreas
Papilloedema – Swelling of the optic disc due to raised intracranial pressure
Papilloma – Benign tumour with a vascular core
Paralytic ileus – Intestinal obstruction due to cessation of peristalsis
Paraplegia – Paralysis of both lower limbs
Parkinson's disease – A degenerative disease associated with tremor and rigidity
Pericardial effusion – Effusion between the two layers of the pericardium
Pericarditis – Inflammation of the pericardium
Peritonitis – Inflammation of the peritoneum
Perthes' disease – Aseptic necrosis of the femoral head epithesis
Petit mal – Epilepsy without major fits
Phlebitis – Inflammation of a vein
Phlebolith – Calcified thrombus within a vein
Placenta praevia – Placenta in an abnormal position
Pleural effusion – Fluid in the pleural cavity
Pleurisy – Inflammation of the pleura
Pneumoconiosis – Lung disease resulting from inhaled dust particles
Pneumonectomy – Surgical removal of a lung
Pneumoperitoneum – The presence of air or gas in the peritoneum
Pneumothorax – The presence of air in the pleural cavity
Poliomyelitis – Inflammation of the grey matter of the spinal cord associated with the poliovirus
Polycythaemia – Increase in the number of red blood cells in the blood
Polydactyly – Congenital presence of extra digits
Polyp – A protuberance of tissue on a stalk
Polyuria – Excessive production of urine
Pott's fracture – Fracture of the lower end of the tibia and fibula
Poupart's ligament – Inguinal ligament
Primigravida – A women pregnant for the first time
Primipara – A woman who has borne her first child
Prolapse – Abnormal descent of a structure within or into a cavity
Prostatectomy – Surgical removal of the prostate gland
Psoriasis – Common skin disease associated with red scaly patches
Pyelonephritis – Inflammation of the pelvis and calyces of the kidney
Pyloric stenosis – A narrowing of the pyloric canal
Pyrexia – A raised temperature associated with a fever

Quadriplegia – Paralysis of all limbs

Rheumatic fever – An infection affecting the heart, valves and the joints
Rheumatoid arthritis – Chronic type of arthritis affecting a number of joints
Rhinorrhoea – Any fluid discharge from the nose
Rickets – Softening and deformity of bone associated with lack of vitamin D in childhood
Rugae – Coarse surface folding (i.e. stomach lining)

Salpingitis – Inflammation of the fallopian tubes
Sarcoidosis – Chronic inflammatory disease of unknown cause
Sarcoma – Malignant tumour arising from connective tissues
Scheurmann's disease – Aseptic necrosis of the vertebral bodies associated with adolescents
Schmorl's node – Bone erosion associated with prolapse of a degenerate intervertebral disc
Sciatica – Pain along the path of the sciatic nerve
Scoliosis – Excessive lateral curvature of the spine
Seminoma – Malignant tumour of the testis associated with younger men
Shingles – A viral disease (chickenpox) of the nervous system
Sinusitis – Inflammation of the nasal accessory sinuses
Spalding's sign – Overlapping of the skull bones indicating fetal death
Spina bifida – Failure of posterior neural arch of a vertebra to develop and unite

Splenomegaly – Enlargement of the spleen
Spondylolisthesis – Forward slipping of L4 or L5 vertebrae due to defect
Spondylosis – Osteoarthritis of the spine
Stenosis – Narrowing of a previously patent passage
Still's disease – Juvenile rheumatoid arthritis
Stricture – Narrowing of a passage
Syndrome – A group of signs and symptoms of disease

Tachycardia – Abnormal rapid heart beat
Tenosynovitis – Inflammation of a tendon sheath
Teratoma – Complex tumour composed of multiple tissues derived from ovary or testis
Tetraplegia – Paralysis of all limbs
Thoracoplasty – Surgical local collapse of the lung by removal of several ribs
Thoracotomy – Surgical opening into the thoracic cavity
Thrombosis – Formation of a clot within a blood vessel
Thrombus – A blood clot
Thyrotoxicosis – Disease associated with overactivity of the thyroid gland
Tinnitus – Noises or ringing in the ears
Torticollis – Twisting of the head to the side associated with spasm of the neck muscles

Ulcer – An open sore of skin or membrane
Uraemia – Symptoms associated with toxic substances in the bloodstream

Valsalva manoeuvre – Forced expiration against a closed glottis
Varices – Dilated veins
Vertigo – Giddiness
Vesical calculus – A bladder stone
Volvulus – Twisting of the bowel obstructing the lumen

Wegener's granuloma – Destructive lesion of nasopharynx – poor prognosis
Whiplash injury – Traumatic injury to cervical spine with acute flexion and extension
Wilms' tumour – A malignant kidney tumour associated with young children

Xerosis – Dryness, often associated with the skin

NORMAL BIOCHEMICAL VALUES

Indicator	Sex	Age	Range	Unit	Comments
Blood urea		<54 >54	2.4–7.0 2.5–8.4	mmol/l mmol/l	Normal dose intravenous urogram ineffective if urea above 10 mmol/l
Serum bilirubin			3.0–20	µmol/l	Oral cholecystography ineffective if above 20 µmol/l
Potassium			3.6–5.0	mmol/l	
Sodium			135–150	mmol/l	
Uric acid	Male Female		250–520 165–400	mmol/l mmol/l	
Erythrocyte sedimentation rate (ESR)	Male Female		0–9 0–15	mm/hour mm/hour	A raised ESR is usually an indication of disease
Bleeding time			3.0–7.0	min	
Clotting time Capillary Venous			 5–7 4–7	 min min	
Blood sugar (fasting)			3.3–6.7	mmol/l	
Cholesterol			<6.0	mmol/l	
Glucose			2.8–8.9	mmol/l	
Calcium			2.1–2.6	mmol/l	
Chloride			95–108	mmol/l	
Bicarbonate			25–35	mmol/l	
Creatinine			45–120	mmol/l	
Albumin			34–50	g/l	
Globulin			16–37	g/l	

COMMON ABBREVIATIONS

AAA	Abdominal Aortic Aneurysm
Ab	Abortion
ACL	Anterior Cruciate Ligament
ADE	Acute Demyelinating Encephalitis
ADH	Antidiuretic Hormone
ADI	Acceptable Daily Intake
ADR	Adverse Drug Reaction
AIDS	Acquired Immune Deficiency Syndrome
ALARA	As Low As Reasonably Achievable
ALLO	Atypical Legionella-like Organisms
AMI	Acute Myocardial Infarction
AML	Acute Myeloid Leukaemia
ARDS	Acute Respiratory Distress Syndrome
ASD	Atrial Septal Defect
ASHD	Arteriosclerotic Heart Disease
ATN	Acute Tubular Necrosis
AVB	Atrioventricular Block
AVH	Acute Viral Hepatitis
AVM	Arteriovenous Malformation
AVR	Aortic Valve Replacement
BBB	Bundle Branch Block
BEL	Breech, Extended Legs
BFL	Breech, Flexed Legs
BI	Bone Injury
BMR	Basal Metabolic Rate
BMT	Bone Marrow Transplant
BO	Bowels Open
BPD	Biparietal Diameter
BPI	Blood Pressure Index
bpm	beats per minute
BSR	Blood Sedimentation Rate
Ca	Carcinoma
CAD	Coronary Artery Disease
CBF	Cerebral Blood Flow
CBP	Chronic Back Pain
CCF	Congestive Cardiac Failure
CDH	Congenital Dislocation of Hip or Coronary Heart Disease
CHF	Congestive Heart Failure
CIBD	Chronic Inflammatory Bowel Disease
CJD	Creutzfeldt-Jakob Disease
COAD	Chronic Obstructive Airways Disease
COPD	Chronic Obstructive Pulmonary Disease
CPB	Cardiopulmonary Bypass
CPR	Cardiopulmonary Resuscitation
CVA	Cerebrovascular Accident
CVP	Central Venous Pressure
DM	Diabetes Mellitus
DOA	Dead On Arrival
DVT	Deep Vein Thrombosis
DXRT	Deep X-ray Therapy

EMI	Elderly with Mental Illness
ERCP	Endoscopic Retrograde Cholangiopancreatography
ESR	Erythrocyte Sedimentation Rate
EUA	Examination Under Anaesthetic
FB	Foreign Body
FFD	Focus-Film Distance
FHR	Fetal Heart Rate
FMNF	Fetal Movements Not Felt
FNA	Fine Needle Aspiration
GBS	Guillain-Barré Syndrome
GHRF	Growth Hormone Releasing Factor
GHIF	Growth Hormone Inhibiting Factor
GOO	Gastric Outlet Obstruction
GIT	Gastrointestinal Tract
GU	Gastric Ulcer
HGH	Human Growth Hormone
HPC	History of Present Complaint
HRT	Hormone Replacement Therapy
IAM	Internal Auditory Meatus
IBD	Inflammatory Bowel Disease
IBS	Irritable Bowel Syndrome
ICP	Intracranial Pressure
IDDM	Insulin Dependent Diabetes Mellitus
IOFB	Intraocular Foreign Body
IOP	Intraocular Pressure
IPH	Intrapartum Haemorrhage
ISD	Interventricular Septal Defect
IUCD	Intrauterine Contraceptive Device
IUD	Intrauterine Death/Device
IVD	Intervertebral Disc
JCA	Juvenile Chronic Arthritis
LAO	Left Anterior Oblique
LBP	Low Back Pain
LFT	Liver Function Test
LLL	Left Lower Lobe
LLO	Legionella-like Organisms
LMP	Last Menstrual Period
LUL	Left Upper Lobe
MABP	Mean Arterial Blood Pressure
MI	Myocardial Infarction
MPAP	Mean Pulmonary Artery Pressure
MR	Mitral Regurgitation
MSU	Mid-Stream Urine
MVD	Mitral Valve Disease
Mx	Mastectomy

NAD	Nil Abnormal Detected	RBBB	Right Bundle Branch Block
NAI	Non-Accidental Injury	RDS	Respiratory Distress Syndrome
NAR	Nasal Airway Resistance	RLL	Right Lower Lobe
NFS	No Fracture Seen	RPN	Renal Papillary Necrosis
NG	New Growth	RTA	Road Traffic Accident
NND	Neonatal Death	RUL	Right Upper Lobe
NWB	Non-Weight Bearing		
		SAH	Subarachnoid Haemorrhage
OA	Osteoarthritis	SDH	Subdural Haemorrhage
OC	Oral Contraceptive	SIDS	Sudden Infant Death Syndrome (Cot
OE	On Examination		Death)
ORIF	Open Reduction Internal	SOL	Space Occupying Lesion
	Fixation		
		TBI	Total Body Irradiation
PCL	Posterior Cruciate Ligament	TKN	Total Knee Replacement
PDA	Patent Ductus Arteriosus	TOF	Tracheo–Oesophageal Fistula
PID	Prolapsed Intervertebral Disc	TSS	Toxic Shock Syndrome
PIH	Pregnancy-Induced Hypertension	TURP	Transurethral Resection of Prostate
PNS	Post Nasal Space	Tx	Transplant
PR	Per Rectum		
PTB	Pulmonary Tuberculosis	URTI	Upper Respiratory Tract Infection
PTE	Pulmonary Thromboembolism	UTI	Urinary Tract Infection
PTRF	Post Transplant Renal Failure		
PUO	Pyrexia of Unknown Origin	VEB	Ventricular Ectopic Beats
PV	Per Vaginam	VLBW	Very Low Birth Weight
PWB	Partial Weight Bearing		
		WB	Weight Bearing
RAS	Renal Artery Stenosis	WBC	White Blood Cell
RB	Recurrent Bleed	WG	Wegener's Granuloma

BIBLIOGRAPHY

Gunn C (2002) *Bones and Joints*, 4th edn. Churchill Livingstone, Edinburgh.

Ionising Radiation (Medical Exposure) Regulations 2000, IR(ME)R 2000 http://www.opsi.gov.uk/si/si2000/20001059.htm

McRae R (2006) *Pocketbook of Orthopaedics and Fractures*, 2nd edn. Churchill Livingstone, Edinburgh.

Raby N, Berman L, de Lacey G (2005) *Accident and Emergency Radiology – A Survival Guide*, 2nd edn. W B Saunders, London.

ELSEVIER CD-ROM LICENCE AGREEMENT

PLEASE READ THE FOLLOWING AGREEMENT CAREFULLY BEFORE USING THIS PRODUCT. THIS PRODUCT IS LICENSED UNDER THE TERMS CONTAINED IN THIS LICENCE AGREEMENT ('Agreement'). BY USING THIS PRODUCT, YOU, AN INDIVIDUAL OR ENTITY INCLUDING EMPLOYEES, AGENTS AND REPRESENTATIVES ('You' or 'Your'), ACKNOWLEDGE THAT YOU HAVE READ THIS AGREEMENT, THAT YOU UNDERSTAND IT, AND THAT YOU AGREE TO BE BOUND BY THE TERMS AND CONDITIONS OF THIS AGREEMENT. ELSEVIER LIMITED ('Elsevier') EXPRESSLY DOES NOT AGREE TO LICENSE THIS PRODUCT TO YOU UNLESS YOU ASSENT TO THIS AGREEMENT. IF YOU DO NOT AGREE WITH ANY OF THE FOLLOWING TERMS, YOU MAY, WITHIN THIRTY (30) DAYS AFTER YOUR RECEIPT OF THIS PRODUCT RETURN THE UNUSED PRODUCT AND ALL ACCOMPANYING DOCUMENTATION TO ELSEVIER FOR A FULL REFUND.

DEFINITIONS As used in this Agreement, these terms shall have the following meanings:

'Proprietary Material' means the valuable and proprietary information content of this Product including without limitation all indexes and graphic materials and software used to access, index, search and retrieve the information content from this Product developed or licensed by Elsevier and/or its affiliates, suppliers and licensors.

'Product' means the copy of the Proprietary Material and any other material delivered on CD-ROM and any other human readable or machine-readable materials enclosed with this Agreement, including without limitation documentation relating to the same.

OWNERSHIP This Product has been supplied by and is proprietary to Elsevier and/or its affiliates, suppliers and licensors. The copyright in the Product belongs to Elsevier and/or its affiliates, suppliers and licensors and is protected by the copyright, trademark, trade secret and other intellectual property laws of the United Kingdom and international treaty provisions, including without limitation the Universal Copyright Convention and the Berne Copyright Convention. You have no ownership rights in this Product. Except as expressly set forth herein, no part of this Product, including without limitation the Proprietary Material, may be modified, copied or distributed in hardcopy or machine-readable form without prior written consent from Elsevier. All rights not expressly granted to You herein are expressly reserved. Any other use of this Product by any person or entity is strictly prohibited and a violation of this Agreement.

SCOPE OF RIGHTS LICENSED (PERMITTED USES) Elsevier is granting to You a limited, non-exclusive, non-transferable licence to use this Product in accordance with the terms of this Agreement. You may use or provide access to this Product on a single computer or terminal physically located at Your premises and in a secure network or move this Product to and use it on another single computer or terminal at the same location for personal use only, but under no circumstances may You use or provide access to any part or parts of this Product on more than one computer or terminal simultaneously.

You shall not (a) copy, download, or otherwise reproduce the Product or any part(s) thereof in any medium, including, without limitation, online transmissions, local area networks, wide area networks, intranets, extranets and the Internet, or in any way, in whole or in part, except for printing out or downloading nonsubstantial portions of the text and images in the Product for Your own personal use; (b) alter, modify, or adapt the Product or any part(s) thereof, including but not limited to decompiling, disassembling, reverse engineering, or creating derivative works, without the prior written approval of Elsevier; (c) sell, license or otherwise distribute to third parties the Product or any part(s) thereof; or (d) alter, remove, obscure or obstruct the display of any copyright, trademark or other proprietary notice on or in the Product or on any printout or download of portions of the Proprietary Materials.

RESTRICTIONS ON TRANSFER This Licence is personal to You, and neither Your rights hereunder nor the tangible embodiments of this Product, including without limitation the Proprietary Material, may be sold, assigned, transferred or sublicensed to any other person, including without limitation by operation of law, without the prior written consent of Elsevier. Any purported sale, assignment, transfer or sublicense without the prior written consent of Elsevier will be void and will automatically terminate the Licence granted hereunder.

TERM This Agreement will remain in effect until terminated pursuant to the terms of this Agreement. You may terminate this Agreement at any time by removing from Your system and destroying the Product and any copies of the Proprietary Material. Unauthorized copying of the Product, including without limitation, the Proprietary Material and documentation, or otherwise failing to comply with the terms and conditions of this Agreement shall result in automatic termination of this licence and will make available to Elsevier legal remedies. Upon termination of this Agreement, the licence granted herein will terminate and You must immediately destroy the Product and all copies of the Product and of the Proprietary Material, together with any and all accompanying documentation. All provisions relating to proprietary rights shall survive termination of this Agreement.

LIMITED WARRANTY AND LIMITATION OF LIABILITY Elsevier warrants that the software embodied in this Product will perform in substantial compliance with the documentation supplied in this Product, unless the performance problems are the result of hardware failure or improper use. If You report a significant defect in performance in writing to Elsevier within ninety (90) calendar days of your having purchased the Product, and Elsevier is not able to correct same within sixty (60) days after its receipt of Your notification, You may return this Product, including all copies and documentation, to Elsevier and Elsevier will refund Your money. In order to apply for a refund on your purchased Product, please contact the return address on the invoice to obtain the refund request form ('Refund Request Form'), and either fax or mail your signed request and your proof of purchase to the address indicated on the Refund Request Form. Incomplete forms will not be processed. Defined terms in the Refund Request Form shall have the same meaning as in this Agreement.

YOU UNDERSTAND THAT, EXCEPT FOR THE LIMITED WARRANTY RECITED ABOVE, ELSEVIER, ITS AFFILIATES, LICENSORS, THIRD PARTY SUPPLIERS AND AGENTS (TOGETHER 'THE SUPPLIERS') MAKE NO REPRESENTATIONS OR WARRANTIES, WITH RESPECT TO THE PRODUCT, INCLUDING, WITHOUT LIMITATION THE PROPRIETARY MATERIAL. ALL OTHER REPRESENTATIONS, WARRANTIES, CONDITIONS OR OTHER TERMS, WHETHER EXPRESS OR IMPLIED BY STATUTE OR COMMON LAW, ARE HEREBY EXCLUDED TO THE FULLEST EXTENT PERMITTED BY LAW.

IN PARTICULAR BUT WITHOUT LIMITATION TO THE FOREGOING NONE OF THE SUPPLIERS MAKE ANY REPRESENTIONS OR WARRANTIES (WHETHER EXPRESS OR IMPLIED) REGARDING THE PERFORMANCE OF YOUR PAD, NETWORK OR COMPUTER SYSTEM WHEN USED IN CONJUNCTION WITH THE PRODUCT, NOR THAT THE PRODUCT WILL MEET YOUR REQUIREMENTS OR THAT ITS OPERATION WILL BE UNINTERRUPTED OR ERROR-FREE.

EXCEPT IN RESPECT OF DEATH OR PERSONAL INJURY CAUSED BY THE SUPPLIERS' NEGLIGENCE AND TO THE FULLEST EXTENT PERMITTED BY LAW, IN NO EVENT (AND REGARDLESS OF WHETHER SUCH DAMAGES ARE FORESEEABLE AND OF WHETHER SUCH LIABILITY IS BASED IN TORT, CONTRACT OR OTHERWISE) WILL ANY OF THE SUPPLIERS BE LIABLE TO YOU FOR ANY DAMAGES (INCLUDING, WITHOUT LIMITATION, ANY LOST PROFITS, LOST SAVINGS OR OTHER SPECIAL, INDIRECT, INCIDENTAL OR CONSEQUENTIAL DAMAGES ARISING OUT OF OR RESULTING FROM: (I) YOUR USE OF, OR INABILITY TO USE, THE PRODUCT; (II) DATA LOSS OR CORRUPTION; AND/OR (III) ERRORS OR OMISSIONS IN THE PROPRIETARY MATERIAL.